Comments on *Positive Action for Health and Wellbeing*
from readers

'I would like to say how much I have benefited from
reading this book. I find it very helpful. This is the first
time since my wife's death that I have actually told
anyone how I feel.'

'Over the years I have read countless self-help books
and none of them helped. I started to read your book and
could identify with most of your clients. No other book
has had this effect on me.'

'Thank you for writing your book. You are helping at
least one human being to make some sense of herself.'

Positive Action for Health and Wellbeing

The practical guide to taking control of your life and your health

Dr Brian Roet

Illustrated by
Shaun Williams

CLASS PUBLISHING • LONDON

Printing history
First published by Macdonald Optima, 1987
Revised edition published by Little, Brown, 1994
Revised edition published by Vermilion, 1996
This edition published by Class Publishing, 2001

The author and publishers welcome feedback from the users of this book.
Please contact the publishers.

Class Publishing (London) Ltd
Barb House, Barb Mews
London W6 7PA
Telephone: 020 7371 2119
Fax: 020 7371 2878
Email: post@class.co.uk
Website: www.class.co.uk

A CIP catalogue record for this book is available from the British Library

ISBN 1 85959 040 3

For details of the rest of Class Publishing's Positive Action
for Health and Wellbeing programme and how to order it,
please see the back of this book.

Positive Action for Health and Wellbeing: The complete step-by-step
programme to take control of your life and your health
ISBN 1 85959 041 1

Positive Action for Health and Wellbeing: Your progress diary
ISBN 1 85959 050 0

Positive Action for Health and Wellbeing: Tape I and Tape II
ISBN 1 85959 042 X

Printed and bound in China

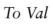

To Val

Acknowledgements

I would like to thank my daughter Danielle who typed the manuscript, a remarkable feat considering my writing is barely decipherable. I would also like to thank the real authors, the patients themselves, who provided case histories, insight and learning and allowed me to be their stenographer.

The illustration on page 93 is reproduced by courtesy of *The Observer*.

Contents

Introduction

Everyone has problems of one kind or another. Some people are able to deal with them and get on with their lives; others become caught up and struggle for years to disentangle themselves. Often this struggle, like the frantic attempt to get out of quicksand, only makes things worse. Constant worry diminishes the enjoyment of life, causing stress and friction in relationships. The more attempts are made to remove the draining distraction, the more the problem and the person become enmeshed.

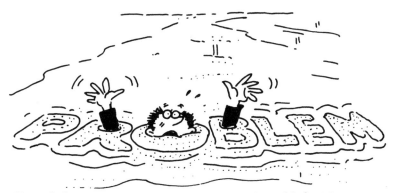

THE STRUGGLE TO DISENTANGLE ONESELF FROM PROBLEMS, LIKE GETTING OUT OF QUICKSAND, OFTEN MAKES THINGS WORSE

How is it that long-term worries are so difficult to resolve? If we bake a cake and it flops, we do not continue to bake inedible cakes; bookshops are full of cookery books to help us out of our plight. Yet there are very few books written in a simple way to help us with far more serious and long-lasting problems.

Intensive studies of prolonged conditions – mental, physical or relationship difficulties – show that the *maintenance of the problem is often related to our attempts to solve it*. Strange though it may seem, what we are doing to overcome the difficulty is actually the cause of its continuation. By directing our attention to this area we may find the key required to solve the problem. Herman Hesse, in his book *Siddhartha*, describes the situation perceptively:

> When someone is seeking it happens quite easily that he only sees the thing he is seeking; that he is unable to find anything, unable to absorb anything because he is only thinking of the thing he is seeking, because he has a goal, because he is obsessed with his goal. Seeking means: to have a goal; but finding means: to be free, to be receptive, to have no goal. You are perhaps indeed a seeker, for in striving towards your goal you do not see many things that are under your nose.

People have chronic troubles in so many areas that it might appear unlikely that a unified approach could be found to resolve them. Yet studying many types of concern shows that there are often common factors related to their maintenance. For ten years Tom has had migraines resistant to a variety of tablets, June has sleep problems not helped by ever-stronger sleeping pills, Pat has chronic constipation unrelieved by laxatives, Suzie is continually struggling with her obesity. How could these diverse conditions have common underlying causes?

The chronic problem has two components – *the problem itself* and *the person involved*. There are also many satellite forces at work, including benefits that may accrue from the problem, the relationships involved, financial factors and so on. They all play a role in the end result. The list of chronic problems is potentially endless, since any unresolved condition will continue until dealt with satisfactorily.

I do not suggest that every medical or relationship problem can be resolved by the methods described in this book. There are obvious situations which require the help of a surgeon or drugs, or which are just unresolvable; but the factors described in the following pages often play a part in many of the conditions that grumble on for year after year.

A list of long-term problems would include obesity, chronic pain, asthma, eczema, phobias, bowel problems, stress-related conditions, marriage difficulties, parent/child problems, addictions such as drugs, cigarettes and alcohol – in fact, to some, life is one big long-term problem.

Attitude may be a major factor in the situation – overprotective spouses, guilty parents, fear of success, fear of failure, all need to be understood to help get the person involved out of a quagmire and back on solid ground. Often people seeking help are hoping for a magic cure – someone else to fix things for them. Unhappily, the magician's wand only exists in fairy tales. Time, effort and responsibility seem to be the main ingredients for change: 'I owe my success to good luck and the harder I work the more luck I seem to have.'

In time, a long-term problem becomes part of the person possessing it – involved in every thought, feeling, work, relationship, benefit and punishment. The longer the problem is enmeshed, the more difficult it is for the person to be without it. Trying to wrest it away forcibly is like tearing off an arm or leg, and just as frightening and painful. This book attempts to look at chronic difficulties from a different angle with the intention of shedding light on the situation by providing a different perspective.

A basic belief threading its way through these pages is that we all play a role in maintaining our troubles and so can learn to play a role in their resolution. An understanding of the components involved in long-term problems and where and how our energies are being misdirected will provide a springboard for change.

This maintenance of problems does not involve conscious malingering with its associated blame and guilt, but a myriad habits and patterns which have become ingrained with time. In order to uncover these perpetuating influences we need to:

- know what to do
- know how to do it
- have support and guidance during the process of change
- make a commitment to provide the necessary effort
- allow time for adjustment.

In this book I hope to provide some of the external requirements needed to release your internal abilities. By gaining insight into the part you are playing in continuing your difficulties, you are then in a better position to do something about them.

My 16-year-old daughter Sophie suffered from herpes (a cold sore) on her lip for many years. Whenever she was worried or in a stressful situation the ugly blemish would appear on her upper lip. Nothing she did seemed to alter the regularity of its appearance, and every few weeks she would show signs of her internal conflict, allowing the virus to gain the upper hand.

A drug company representative informed me of a powerful new cream, which would prevent cold sores if applied early enough. I told Sophie about this new cream and bought some for her. She was very eager to try it and told her school friends about her discovery. She never in fact used the cream, but since then there has been no sign of a cold sore; apparently her change of attitude provided her body with a defence mechanism, which overcame the virus without help from the cream.

There are many reports of cases where altered attitudes, relaxation, increased confidence or visualization (looking at internal pictures) have played a major role in breaking the cycle of chronic suffering; these results are not random, and an underlying logic provides the basis for untangling the problem. As each person is unique, their troubles will also have individual characteristics. To gain from this book, it is important to understand the general principles and translate them into your own personal situation. Chronic problems become ensnared in every aspect of one's life; so proceeding slowly and cautiously will help you to build up confidence along the way.

There *is* a choice available, although this is often not apparent to the chronic sufferer; by learning more about yourself you will increase the energy and drive available to make small changes. Even taking small steps up a steep mountainside means that progress is being made and can be measured by the changing scenery, which offers proof that the challenge is being overcome.

Inevitably, pitfalls and setbacks will occur along the way; by learning from these and continuing to work at the problem, progress can be maintained. Often the breakthrough comes by doing something differently, as in the following case.

Geraldine, a shy, retiring 50-year-old, has lacked confidence for most of her life. At work she is usually the first to arrive, but she has to wait outside until someone comes with the key. She has asked for a key on several occasions over a three-year period, but has never received one; often she has shivered in the rain and snow waiting for someone to let her in.

Encouraged by friendly colleagues to begin standing up for herself, she came to see me. Gradually, her self-confidence grew and she decided to do something about it. She declared that if she were not given a key she would arrive late the next day. That evening she had still not received a key, so she made the difficult and (for her) frightening decision to arrive late the following morning. The next day she waited at home, feeling nervous and guilty, wondering what would be said when she walked in late. That evening she was presented with a key.

Geraldine's problem may sound simple to most of us, but our problems are often simple when viewed by others; it required much courage and anxiety for Geraldine to make that positive stand. Whenever we alter our actions we fear terrible things may result; generally, they don't.
This book is about the possibility of taking suitable chances, making different decisions, achieving altered attitudes. In order to break free from the circle of misery, risks may have to be taken and experiences be undergone. The

worst that can happen is that we learn something new; the best is that a partial solution may begin to appear, presenting us with our key to the future.

In my practice, a major factor in helping clients is giving them time and listening to their concerns with a supportive ear. All the techniques in the world will fail if the client is not supported in the process of change. Time is also an essential ingredient for change – time for change to occur and quiet time, necessary for the client on a daily basis.

There is advice in this book that can help to improve your perspective on life. Your task, as the reader, is to find advice that is suitable for you and to put time and effort into using it.

To make the most of the book, don't flip through it, or read it like a novel. Take one chapter at a time. Use the *Progress Diary* to help you digest what you have read and to think about how it could be applied to you and any problem you may have.

PART 1

Basic components

1

The long-term problem

'It is more important to know what sort of person has a disease than to know what sort of disease a person has.'
Hippocrates

Life is a maze in which we take the wrong turning before we have learned to walk. Long-term problems can be viewed from four different perspectives:

- *Accepting things as they are.* You learn to live with the problem, accepting that a small amount of energy and enjoyment will be drained away by it, but realizing that this is the price to be paid and getting on with the rest of your life in the best possible way.
- *Attempting to solve the problem.* You try to fix it and remove it completely. This requires effort, time and responsibility; you need to be prepared for hopes to be raised and dashed, for frustrations and successes, dead-ends and freeways, with a mind open to learning along the way.
- *Recognizing the problem as a message.* You see it as a

means of understanding yourself emotionally or within relationships. By various methods explained in this book, you may learn how to acknowledge your feelings, how emotions such as fear and guilt are intertwined with your suffering and how to gain benefits from the predicament you are in. This means understanding the cry for help at one level, and the maintenance of the *status quo* at another.

- *Using avoidance and denial* to ensure a circular motion of non-progress. In this way any helpful advice can be blocked or ignored in a multitude of ways – deferring, forgetting, 'yes-but'ing, using pseudo-logic to maintain the situation as it is and seeking answers elsewhere.

ACCEPTING THE SITUATION

'A problem is a matter difficult of settlement or solution.'
Chambers' 20th Century Dictionary

Once upon a time, in a small Polish village, the inhabitants were constantly complaining. Some moaned that their houses were too small, others because they were too poor. Some complained about their wives, others that they had none. The wise man of the village, growing sick and tired of all the problems, summoned the villagers to a meeting in the market square. He asked them all to go home and write their complaints on a piece of paper, and to return the next day. They did as he requested, and returned to find he had erected a tree in the centre of the square.

'This is a problem tree,' he told them. 'I want each of you to tie your problems to the branches of the tree.' They followed his instructions and soon hundreds of pieces of paper were fluttering in the breeze.

'Now I would like you, one at a time, to go around the

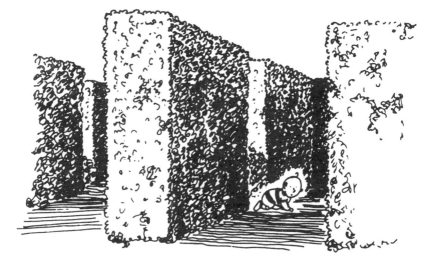

LIFE IS A MAZE IN WHICH WE TAKE THE WRONG
TURNING BEFORE WE HAVE LEARNED TO WALK.

tree reading the problems, and to choose the one you would most like to have.' One after the other, the villagers trooped round the tree, perused the writings, and removed the problem which they most wanted to have. At the end of the day they all found they had chosen their own problem.

In any situation where someone claims there is a problem it is essential to discover:

- if there really is a problem;
- if so, *who* has the problem.

Some people complain about situations that are unchangeable facts of life. These are not 'matters difficult of solution', but situations that are inevitable and unresponsive to change. Parents, for example, complain about the 'problems' they have with their teenage children and sometimes are driven to seek professional advice. They complain that the children do not tidy their rooms, dress properly, are late for meals, smoke, are not polite to adults, stay out late, and so on.

Once these are seen as problems, much time, energy and emotion is spent trying to resolve them. Hours are spent in discussion, worry, reasoning, bribery, punishment, all ·to solve a problem which may be a natural phenomenon of growing up. The sleepless nights and grey hairs, as a rule, have no marked effect on the behaviour of the teenagers involved.

If this behaviour can be seen as temporary, common and perhaps useful, then it may be easier to accept. This may not make it any more pleasant for the parents, but at least it is not viewed as a problem to solve, but as a transient difficulty to be lived with and understood.

In a Jewish village a man kept complaining about his house and household. His friends became tired of the constant moaning and suggested he see a rabbi and ask for his help. The man went to the rabbi and for some hours bemoaned his fate. He rambled on about his house being too small, his furniture old, his wife not pretty, his children untidy ... etc. The rabbi listened patiently and when the moaner had finished claimed that he could help. The man was delighted and eagerly asked what he should do to overcome his immense problems.

'Buy a goat', replied the rabbi gently.

'Whatever for?' gasped the astounded man.

'Don't ask questions. You came to me with a problem. I'm the wise man. Trust me and buy the goat.'

A week later the confused man returned to the rabbi dragging a small brown goat on a string.

'Good,' said the rabbi. 'Now go and tether the goat on a long string in your house. No questions, just do as I say and return in a week.'

Slowly and with a bewildered expression, the man led the goat home. A week later he returned, dishevelled, smelly and looking very tired.

'The goat is destroying my house. He eats everything in sight, messes all over the place, makes a terrible noise and smells awful. My wife and children are at their wits' end and think I have gone mad. Please help me.'

'Good,' said the rabbi. 'Now go and sell the goat and return to see me in a week.'

A week later the man returned neat, fresh and smiling.

'How are things?' inquired the rabbi.

'Wonderfully peaceful,' the man replied. 'My house is now my home, clean and tidy, and my wife and children are very happy. Thank you for your help!'

Some people, like the moaner in this story, are disciples of the commandment 'Life should be fair!' As they grew up they were told either directly or indirectly that things would turn out according to some unseen moral justice.

The fact is life is *not* fair, it never has been and is unlikely to be so in the future. One only needs to read the papers to notice all the injustice which is continually heaped on the huge majority of the world's population. Those who believe that life should be fair face a vast number of problems. Whenever fate deals an unpleasant blow, it is seen as a problem that should not have occurred and to which there *must* be an answer. Complaining it is not fair and waiting for someone else to fix it is like waiting for a bus halfway between bus stops.

There is considerable truth in the old cliché that 'the problem is not the problem, it is the *worry about it* that is the problem.' For many sufferers of long-term problems it is this worry that keeps the wheel of the problem turning, whereas some understanding or acceptance of the situation might allow resolution to occur and would certainly save a lot of wasted energy.

Five-year-old Suzie wets her bed. Suzie and her Mum came to see me because of this problem. Suzie's elder sister Jackie stopped wetting the bed when she was three. Ever since Suzie turned three, Mum has tried to find a solution to *her* problem. She has worried, discussed with Dad, neighbours and school teachers, consulted doctors and had long talks with Suzie, all to no avail.

Both Suzie and Mum are caught up with nocturnal and morning rituals to deal with 'the problem'. Suzie is not allowed to drink after 6 pm, is sat on the toilet for 10 minutes before bed and picked up during the night. In the morning the sheets are examined and any improvement, or otherwise, discussed. Dad, kept informed of the situation, entered into the debate with praise or criticism.

In my opinion, the problem was not with Suzie and the bedwetting, but with Mum's *worrying* and comparison to elder sister Jackie. I felt Mum was prolonging the situation by her worry and attempts to solve a 'non problem'. Had she been able to accept the fact that her two daughters were different and so were developing differently, the chances are that Suzie would not still be wetting her bed.

In any problem (or non problem) situation, assessing *who* has the problem is of the utmost relevance. Doctors recognize this and talk about the 'identified patient', inferring that the person thrust forward as having the problem has been identified by others but, in fact, may not be the patient. This is often the case with children brought in with behavioral

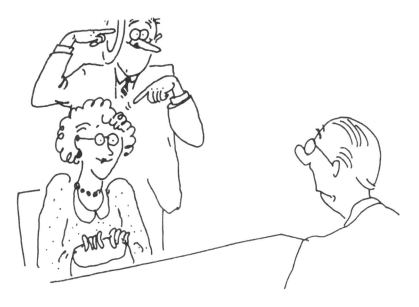

IT IS IMPORTANT TO RECOGNISE WHO HAS THE PROBLEM ...

problems. It becomes obvious after a short while that the child would benefit if the parents received help.

To decide who actually has the problem one should note *who* is complaining. The person complaining is the one with the problem even though it may appear that the one being complained about *should* have the problem.

'Could you please stop my wife smoking, it is driving me mad', really means the husband has a problem but is not seeking help for it.

'My little boy won't eat his meals properly. Please tell him he will not grow up properly if he doesn't eat all his vegetables.' How difficult it is to help such mothers realize who has the problem.

Many people worry about the problems of others. 'I'm so worried about my son-in-law's attitude to my daughter. He doesn't treat her correctly and I lay awake all night thinking about it. I need help to get to sleep and not be so anxious.'

People like these are 'problem thieves'. They steal other people's problems and are constantly worried about what they can do, when they can do nothing at all to help the situation. Many parents fall into this category because of their love of and concern for their children. Unfortunately, it is the other person's problem, and if they cannot or will not deal with it, 'stealing' it from them does not help. The worrier is merely wasting energy that could be used more positively in other aspects of their life.

ATTEMPTING TO SOLVE THE PROBLEM

'If we can really understand the problem
the answer will come out of it,
because the answer is not separate from the problem.'
Krishnamurti

Research at a therapy clinic in California has shown that a high proportion of treatment failures were the result of an inadequate definition of the problem during the first visit. Mrs Beeton echoed this when, in her recipe for jugged hare, she wrote: 'First catch the hare'.

It is vitally important to define the problem before treatment begins to see if it is a real problem capable of solution and, if so, what solution would be acceptable. Seeking help for a problem of the 'I want to be happy' sort is futile and a waste of time.

Many patients describe their problems in such vague and nebulous terms that a solution is almost impossible.

- I can't cope with things!
- I'm being hooked into the situation!

- I'm so depressed.
- I just feel lousy all the time.

These descriptions need to be analyzed in greater detail, to be pared down to the essentials before a pathway comes into sight for resolution. The first step is to ask yourself questions such as:

- what does it mean to me?
- how does it feel?
- what limits my dealing with it?
- what role does my attitude play?

Once the basic components are understood it becomes possible to begin to correct things.

Most of us approach the problem on a logical basis – I have this pain, there must be a cause, a physical reason, with all the advances of modern medicine an answer must be found. The various ports of call on this journey are the doctor, the hospital, tablets, tests, specialists, further tests, stronger tablets, different treatment, advice from the multitude; the ocean between is littered with anger, frustration, disappointment, fear, guilt and hopelessness.

Sometimes an answer is found, the problem is resolved and life takes an upturn where optimism and energy return and external events can be enjoyed and appreciated, leaving the problem behind as a nasty experience. But resolution often involves different attitudes, approaching things on a different level, viewing the situation from a distance rather than being engulfed by it. People rigid in their attitudes find it difficult to influence the problem for which they are seeking relief. Being fixed, inflexible and unable to incorporate new opinions will ensure the merry-go-round continues.

It is necessary to put time and effort into making the desired changes. Sufferers frequently voice the desire to make the changes, but their actions or attitudes convey a different message.

'I'm so overweight I can't get into any of my clothes. I need help and will do *anything* to lose weight.'

'Do you realize you will have to eat less?'

'But I can't doctor. I love my food so much I couldn't possibly eat any less than I do.'

'My husband and I argue continually and I'm frightened he will leave me. What can I do?'

'Let's analyze what is happening between the two of you and see where you can change what you are doing.'

'But I *can't* change doctor, I've always been the way I am and it's too late to change me now.'

It is obvious that if a long-term problem exists it is mostly likely to be resolved by an alteration in attitude, thought or action. Continue to behave in exactly the same way and nothing will change.

One of the difficulties about changing a situation is the inertia caused by being in that predicament for some time. It requires energy to make a decision and do something different; it is much easier to continue along the same old path, however many potholes are present; it is easier to *hope* that things will get better than to do something to ensure that they do.

To alter a problem you need to be:

- irritated by the suffering;
- eager for change and believe change is possible;
- prepared to accept responsibility for change and have an open attitude towards alternatives;

- confident to try something new and committed to doing so;
- aware of what to do and how to do it.

RECOGNIZING THE PROBLEM AS A MESSAGE

'Problems are only opportunities in disguise.'

Viewing difficulties as opportunities to learn provides a completely new slant on the situation. This attitude, however, requires a suitable level of maturity; telling a screaming child who has just tumbled off a bike that this is part of the process of learning to ride is unlikely to achieve the desired response. Many people are not sufficiently adult in their emotions to accept their suffering as an opportunity to learn about themselves.

One of the most prevalent and restricting attitudes towards chronic problems is not facing up to them or acknowledging the various factors involved. By turning towards the difficulty and accepting it as something to learn from, another train of thought begins, allowing gradual but definite erosion of the problem.

If we analyzed our early life we would find many unpleasant incidents that, in fact, had enabled us to learn things about ourselves, our abilities or those around us.

Recently, while travelling to a destination in the country I decided on a new route off the motorway. The inevitable happened; I became hopelessly lost and was frustrated, perplexed and anxious. However, during attempts to rediscover the correct road I found something in an antique shop I'd been seeking for years, a really nice pub and a stately home which I intend to revisit. But, and this is important, I was able to acknowledge the opportunity that being lost presented to me.

If, instead of trying to solve the problem and remove it, we ask ourselves 'what does it mean, what message is involved, what can I learn from it?', we will follow a completely different pathway, often with pleasantly surprising results.

Jeremy had suffered chest pains for years. He tried to diagnose and remove it by physical means – ECGs, chest X-rays and tablets – to no avail. The 'try to cure it' routine was not working. I asked him if he would accept the pain as part of life's problems but he was unwilling to do so.

I then suggested we try to learn from the pain and he agreed to spend time and effort following that course. We analyzed the pain: when it occurred, what effect it had on him, any benefits to him or his family, things that made it worse or better, how he would be if it was not part of him.

After discussing the various aspects of his condition we summarized it:

- he had suffered the pain on and off for 10 years;
- it occurred when he was feeling relaxed, calm and happy;
- there was a strong underlying guilt about being illegitimate and a feeling he had caused enormous problems for his mother;
- he had a very low opinion of himself, no confidence and a belief he had been responsible for the vagrancy of his son and the failed marriage of his daughter.

I asked him to 'go inside' the pain by focusing his mind internally on it and then let any messages drift into his mind. He sat motionless with his eyes closed for some minutes then silent tears started to roll down his cheeks. In his pain he saw pictures of himself as a small boy being called 'a bastard' and having to fight for survival. He also saw hordes of adults accusing him of a multitude of mishaps and sufferings.

After he settled down we discussed what he had learnt from the pain. He said 'It seems as if the pain is acting to punish me for what I have done; it is also isolating me from others so I can't hurt them and perhaps it is helping me receive the sympathy and attention I've never had.'

Jeremy was on a path of learning from his pain and we discussed how he could go about using that knowledge to grow, become more confident and face the world without feeling guilty or requiring punishment. As he incorporated that advice and understanding his confidence grew and the need for the pain diminished.

USING AVOIDANCE AND DENIAL

'Denial of the real problem may in fact be the real problem.'

Recently I caught a plane to Australia. I checked in my luggage and the attendant weighed the suitcase, attaching a luggage label for Melbourne. The thread on the label broke and she cursed and attached another which also broke.

'These label strings are faulty, they are all breaking', she remarked as she tried to attach a third label. My mind drifted to the millions of pounds spent by the airline on advertising services, food and so on which were going to end up with a dissatisfied customer – all because of faulty string costing almost nothing. I imagined how annoyed tourists would be to arrive in Australia and find that their luggage was in Bombay; I also thought about the trouble and expense needed to unite the two.

I asked the girl why she didn't get some more suitable string. She replied that there was some at another counter but she couldn't be bothered to get it. I made sure my label wasn't attached with the faulty thread.

Many people in unpleasant circumstances continually *talk* about how difficult things are but never do anything about them.

'I'm so fed up with John leaving dirty ashtrays around the house.'
'Why don't you tell him about it?'
'I will one day but it is just so annoying.'

Perhaps the continual discussion of the problem in some way relieves the tension. Maybe people may not want to change but get benefit from the constant grumbling.

'These headaches have been driving me mad for years. I take so many tablets I must be rattling.'
'Why don't you see a doctor?'
'I keep meaning to but I never have the time. I'm sure they will stop soon but they are such a nuisance.'

Endeavours to solve long-term difficulties require initiative and persistence to arrive at a suitable solution. Many attempts are fraught with failure; doors that seem to open easily lead to dead ends further ahead. Conflicting advice from friends makes matters worse. In the long run it is really up to us. It is our problem, unique to us and only we can fully understand it.

There are those who cart their suffering around believing either that there is nothing wrong or that, by avoiding it, it will go away. Any attempts to help them confront what is happening is resisted. There are excuses, deferrals and a multitude of other avoidance tactics.

Such people guarantee their life membership on the merry-go-round of long-term problems, never prepared to place their feet on firm ground and face what is causing all the trouble. By so doing they drag many others along for the ride, all those 'do-gooders' who believe they can help are initially taken in by complaints about the situation, pleas for assistance, sympathy and pity. It is only after they have been dragged around and around for ages that realization dawns – enough is enough, and managing to overcome their guilt they break free.

To provide the best basis for change we need to sift through the vast quantities of advice and comparisons thrust our way, turn a deaf ear to those who seem in no position to guide us, and build our stepping stones slowly and cautiously according to our own pace to arrive at the safety of the other side.

TURNING POINTS

1 Define the problem accurately.
2 Recognize if it is a real problem or a non problem.
3 Understand *who* has the problem.
4 Enumerate what measures you have already tried to solve the problem.
5 Consider whether acceptance might not be a suitable solution.
6 Look at attempts to solve the problem which may actually be maintaining it.
7 Make a commitment to put time and effort in the right direction to improve the situation.
8 Face up to the problem rather than avoiding or denying it.
9 Consider carefully if the problem is a message – the best alternative available for the time being (see page 12).
10 Analyze what strengths or abilities you require to overcome the problem and live without it.

2

The Patient

People on the never-ending circuit, constantly attempting to resolve their long-term problems, often have characteristics relevant to their position. Examining these traits may help us understand how they got on to the merry-go-round and why they are unable to dismount from it.

Many long-term patients have repeatedly followed incorrect advice and are naturally very wary or 'resistant' to any further attempts at help. They cling desperately to their own personal knowledge as the only safety they have experienced. Consciously they are anxious and willing to change and accept alternatives, but unconscious fear prevents them getting off the merry-go-round.

'This pain I've been having for years is killing me. Please help me doctor.'

'If you try relaxation and self-hypnosis it may be a good start to lessen the tension.'

'I'll try *anything* if it will relieve the pain.'

'Good. Just practise these exercises every day and I'll see you in a week.'

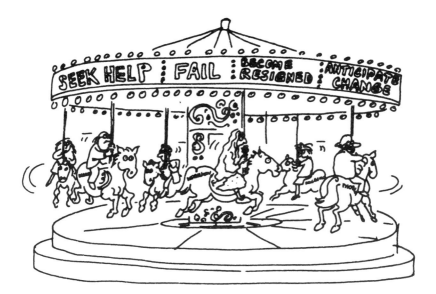

A week later:

'How did you get on with the exercises?'
'I just couldn't do them. There was so much going on in our house I couldn't find a moment to rest. The pain is still killing me doctor, what can I do?'

The conscious affirmation 'I'll try *anything*' is real and fully intended, but the old treadmill of habit takes control and the best intentions lose impetus.

A wise therapist once said that the first step in any attempt to be of use was 'to be where the patient is. Start with his attitudes and beliefs and gradually lead him in a more beneficial direction from *his* starting point, not yours.'

Riding a horse along a country road you hear galloping hooves behind you. Turning round you see a runaway horse approaching. You spur your horse on to a gallop and grab hold of the panicking horse's bridle. You have two choices – come to a sudden halt to stop the horse or continue on at its own pace for a while, gradually slowing down and easing it to the side of the road.

Patients with long-term problems are like the unwary horse. They are rushing in a direction they are unsure of, caught in the insecurity of the prolonged discomfort, desperately seeking help but unable to be abruptly halted and turned in a different direction. They resist any excess pressure so that anyone offering help needs to be gentle, supporting and have untiring patience while gradually offering alternative choices.

The unfortunate aspect of such patients' plight is that the more they twist and turn to free themselves the more they become entangled. Each time another ray of hope is extinguished they realize there may be *no* real solution to the problem and the ensuing battle-weariness adds further difficulties. These repeated failures increase the sensitivity to the patients' 'failure antennae' so that they give up more easily each time they try something new. The passage of time only makes matters worse as energy and hope are slowly drained by experience.

For many years June had had problems with sleeping. She saw me out of desperation and during the first session I made a tape which would help her relax and drift off to sleep. When she returned a week later she complained that although she had slept better she still had some bad nights and felt this form of treatment was sure to fail. Her warning 'antennae' were so sensitive that she anticipated failure long before a suitable assessment was possible. Her past experiences had made her so aware of the possibility of failure that she was eager to grasp it as an answer.

THE DANGERS OF MISUNDERSTANDING

One of the most common complaints of the long-term sufferer is a feeling of not being understood, either by friends, relatives or the medical profession. This misunderstanding often results from the extreme difficulty of 'being in the other person's shoes'. It is hard to understand difficulties and restrictions if you 'haven't been there yourself'. All too often we think, feel and comment in a way relating to how *we* would act with the condition, but unless we put ourselves in the patients' place we will find it extremely difficult to understand them.

I was on a crowded train in Melbourne years ago and someone behind me trod on my heel. I winced in pain and ignored it. A few minutes later the same thing happened and I felt my anger rise. I asked myself, why doesn't that so and so look where he's standing, how unthoughtful people are and if it happened again I would turn around and give him a piece of my mind. A few minutes later I again got a searing pain in my heel as he stood on it a third time. I wheeled around, my anger about to burst forth, until I saw the person responsible – it was an elderly blind man. My failure to appreciate his problem led to my anger.

This lack of understanding, whether real or imagined, can cause immense problems, particularly if the patient is visiting a doctor who, after all, is trained to make people better and, by implication, to understand their problems. Any look or reaction on the doctor's part is interpreted as a sign of disbelief. 'You think I'm imagining it doctor, don't you?' is a common question, and no amount of reassurance will help. The added frustration of being regarded as a malingerer only makes matters worse.

People are labelled as moaners, whiners, hypochondriacs, and in time the label sticks. Yet the questions, doubts, fears and symptoms are *real* and desperately need understanding. It is very rewarding to see the face of a patient who has at last been understood by a sympathetic listener; it is as if sharing the problem has halved it.

THE PATIENT'S DILEMMA

Most chronic sufferers feel angry, often with good reason. After months and years of discomfort an answer still has not been found so anger builds up at the doctor, themselves, the world. Anger directed at the medical profession, results from the multiple failures or extra problems resulting from the treatment received. The false underlying belief that there *must* be an answer, a solution, a cure, causes much anger when this is not achieved. But just as a child dependent on its parents finds it difficult to be angry with them, so it is with patient and doctor. How can you be angry with the doctors when they are your only hope of salvation? But, nevertheless, you *are* angry with the doctors.

An acute dilemma faces long-term patients: they are continually seeking advice yet are in no suitable position to receive or judge it. They are constantly reminded by the symptom that something is wrong and a remedy must be found – but what? Doctors often don't have enough time for explanations and may use prescriptions or tests to avoid a confrontation.

A doctor taking a history from a patient had the following conversation:

Doctor: 'How old are you Mrs Jones?'
Patient: 'Fifty.'

Doctor: 'Are your parents still alive?'
Patient: 'Mum is, but Dad died five years ago.'
Doctor: 'What did he die from?'
Patient: 'I don't know, but the doctors said it was nothing serious.'

On another occasion I had to give an anaesthetic to a patient who was to have her kidney removed. Talking to her the night before the operation I asked her why she was having her kidney removed. She replied that she had no idea. 'When the doctor examined me and arranged the operation he was in such a hurry I didn't dare ask.'

Sadly such stories are not unique and are damaging to doctors and patients alike.

WHAT MAKES A LONG-TERM PATIENT?

Are there any basic characteristics about long-term patients which may play a role in maintaining their condition? Are some weaknesses allowing a symptom or situation to be prolonged: Could a similar situation be resolved more rapidly by someone of a different personality?

In attempting to build an 'Identikit' picture, I am, of course, working with generalities, so don't be surprised if a long-term sufferer who you know, whether yourself, a relative or friend, does not fit the picture completely. Remember, too, that the characteristics described may be a *cause* or *result* of the condition, and that no moralistic judgment is as helpful as a basic understanding of the person concerned. The long-term patient may be suffering from any complaint, and what we are trying to do is to establish whether such patients have characteristics in common which may explain why they have their chronic conditions.

The following lengthy list of characteristics is based on my experience of treating long-term patients:

- the complaint first occurred many months or years ago. The condition will have fluctuated in intensity, often for no apparent reason;
- help will have been sought on many occasions from multiple sources – the medical profession, alternative therapies, neighbours, magazines;
- the patient's hopes will have been raised and dashed many times;
- the patient continues to seek help although by now is pessimistic of any resolution;
- the patient's family and colleagues are well aware when the condition is worse, because of changes in attitude and mood swings;
- beneath the surface of everyday life there is a considerable degree of anger and when this surfaces it is directed at friends or relations;
- frustration is another factor, the patient frequently asking 'Why me?';
- the patient lacks confidence and is pessimistic not only about the outcome, but about daily situations;
- the patient needs much support and understanding from close family and friends, and repeated reassurance that things will get better;
- there are periods of fear or panic that nothing will ever change;
- there is a personality change as the condition erodes the patient's original, more carefree nature;
- although constantly seeking an answer 'out there', the patient prefers to avoid self-analysis of the role he or she is playing in maintaining the condition;
- the patient is very resistant to any suggestion that there

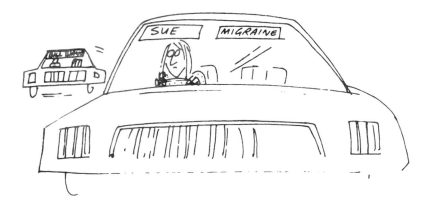

may be a psychological element in the problem, prefer-
ring to look for a physical cause and physical treatment
and avoiding any psychological therapy (see page
121);
- the patient has bouts of depression when all hope seems
  lost and everything looks gloomy;
- the tablets the patient is taking have minimal benefits.
  They may also have side effects and have led to
  dependency;
- the patient continually talks, discusses and analyzes the
  problem with anyone who will listen, and uses semi-
  medical terms gleaned over the years;
- the patient often blames another person or situation for
  the condition rather than taking the responsibility for
  it;
- constant involvement with the problem vastly diminishes the patient's ability to enjoy life;
- a 'system' has developed with other members of the
  family in which each plays a role to accommodate the
  condition and thus prolong it;
- there is often an element of underlying guilt and fear;

- there may be unconscious benefits from the condition which are unrecognized but are factors in maintaining the problem (see page 42);
- the doctor regards the patient as resistant or neurotic, which only adds to the frustration, anger and guilt;
- there have been many occasions when the treatment made the condition worse;
- feelings of hopelessness and anticipation of success constantly battle in the patient's mind;
- although continuing to seek an answer, the patient is resigned that there is none;
- the patient cannot accept the condition as part of himself or herself;
- the patient joins the 'club' of long-term sufferers alongside others in a similar situation who understands the problem (see pages 110–111);
- the merry-go-round of seeking help, failing, becoming resigned, then anticipating change, becomes ingrained in the patient's personality as he or she becomes labelled a 'chronic patient';
- in time the patient identifies with the condition, which becomes part of him or her;
- the condition acts as a form of punishment, either of the patient or of someone close;
- the condition may provide an excuse or justification for particular behaviour or failure in certain aspects of life; a sense of humour is often missing because of the energy drained away by the chronic problem.

TURNING POINTS

1 If you have a long-term problem it is likely that
   you are unconsciously playing a major role in
   maintaining your problem.
2 Understanding yourself – attitudes, beliefs, feelings
   – will allow you to be in a better position to
   deal with your problem.
3 Do not blame yourself or see yourself as a
   malingerer or as intentionally hanging on to your
   problem.
4 Recognize that your energy may have been
   drained by the long-term condition you have.
5 Find a suitable understanding person to share
   your beliefs and advise you in a supportive way.
6 Take responsibility for your problem and for its
   resolution.
7 Check the 'Identikit' list to note how many
   descriptions are relevant to you.

The need for a symptom

Love Your Disease – it's keeping you healthy
Title of book by Dr John Harrison

'As long as humans feel threatened and helpless,
they will seek the sanctuary that illness provides.'
Dr T. Rynearson, *Journal of Clinical Psychiatry*

LEARNING BY EXPERIENCE

We learn from experience – our own experience. We may
listen to advice but usually it is the *practical application* of
that advice which enables us to learn and maintain the new
learning as a positive memory.

When confronted by a new situation, previous experiences enable us to deal with it effectively. We rapidly check
any stored knowledge to make use of the details to gain
confidence and proceed in an appropriate way.

The art of growing up involves the confrontation of
thousands of new situations about which we have no prior
knowledge. We use our limited experience, a desire to

change and the courage to take risks, to help us deal with these new experiences.

It could be said that requirements for growth are:

- an inner force or desire for change;
- the ability to take risks – courage to attempt something new;
- access to talents or experience which might be helpful;
- the strength to overcome the pain of mistakes made during a transition period;
- an internal alteration to the learning pattern enabling us to react differently to future situations.

If you have ever watched a baby learning to walk, you will understand the processes involved in this change. Initially, the baby crawls about quite happily, apart from the occasional painful bump, seeing the world from a safe and familiar vantage point.

Then an innate force, guided by parental encouragement, impels the baby to stand upright. The world suddenly looks unfamiliar, the baby wobbles, falls down and bursts into tears. This experience is the beginning. Gradually, after many falls and much support, the baby learns to stand upright unaided. Then, with more practice and growing confidence, standing will become an automatic process and there will be no need to go through the mistakes and learning process every time the child wishes to stand up.

In my opinion learning from experience is one of the greatest demarcations between those who make positive changes with time and those who continue with long-term repetitive patterns of behaviour.

So many people complaining about difficulties are not

able to learn from positive experiences. They ignore, deny
or misread anything good that happens to them:

'It was just a coincidence.'
'I only won because everyone else was no good.'
'I only got the job because they liked my suit.'

Many and varied excuses are used to avoid taking
responsibility for positive experiences.

One 25-year-old girl, Josephine, was unable to accept
any positive action that she did. Her fear was that
admitting this would lead her away from 'the safety of
failure'. She had a fear of travelling on buses and felt she
would panic and have to get off the bus.

After much discussion she agreed to go on a bus trip
where she could get off and change buses as many times as
she liked. Her aim was to complete the journey, even if it
took all day, and learn from the experience.

When I saw her the following week she was in a low
mood and I assumed she had been unable to complete the
journey. When I asked her what had happened, she replied:

'Oh, I did the journey in one bus. I didn't panic at all.'
    'You must be delighted,' I said.
    'No. I don't feel any different. I did the journey on a
Sunday so it doesn't count.'

Josephine was able to deny *anything* that may be
regarded as positive behaviour on her part. Her life was a
stalemate. She made no progress. She added no valuable
experience as time passed by. It wasn't that she was just
pessimistic, she was unable to use her life events to build
strength and confidence.

If we can find positive experiences we develop more

choices, hence are less frightened by what confronts us (see Ch. 24 – Panning for Gold). If we develop an attitude of 'What can I learn?' rather than 'Is it a success or a failure?' we are freer to embark on new experiences with less fear of blame or guilt. Most of our learning in life comes from mistakes, so it follows that the more mistakes we make the more learned we become.

Often there is a voice inside saying? 'Better the devil you know than the one you don't. Stay where you are – it may be uncomfortable but at least you know it's safe; if you do something new you never know where that may lead you.' This voice needs to be challenged and overcome. If you listen to it life will pass you by.

By standing still as time moves on you are actually drifting backwards.

HOW THE SYMPTOMS DEVELOP

This pattern continues as we grow up and develop. The human body and mind may be viewed as a compact package of potential. It has in store immense mental and physical powers which are waiting to be liberated. Throughout a lifetime, a person will endeavour to release this potential to achieve a major proportion of what is available. If pain or fear occur during the learning process we may instinctively restrict our growth in that direction, so developing limitations in later life. As we learn from experience, frightening or severely painful experiences will teach us the benefits of avoidance.

If a situation is too painful to accept, we may substitute a symptom rather than dealing with the challenge. This symptom provides initial benefits, perhaps of avoidance, but as time, and the initial challenge, passes, the need for the symptom is no longer appropriate. However, it has

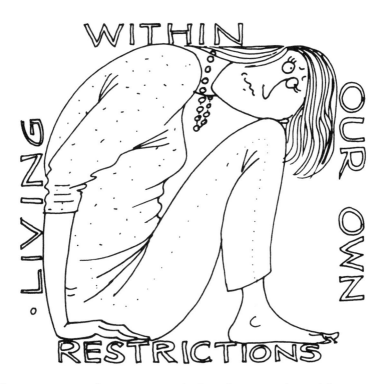

become part of our 'repertoire' and so remains with us.

It is as if there are two ways of dealing with an awkward situation. We can use an appropriate ability developed by experimental learning as we grew, or if this is unavailable, a symptom may be a suitable unconscious substitute. The symptom is provided by the unconscious mind to avoid pain, fear and guilt and is not initiated as a malicious or devious method of avoidance.

In the early stages the symptom is essential and compensates us for losing the ability to deal with things any other way. In turn a habit develops incorporating the symptom and even though the 'danger zone' was passed many years earlier, the force of habit perpetuates the symptom.

It's as if a learner driver nearly had an accident and, as a result of fear, drives at less than the required speed. Over the next few years his or her driving ability improves but the by now redundant fear still causes over-cautious driving, creating problems for the driver and other road users.

THE BENEFITS OF SYMPTOMS

'Suffering makes us neither good nor bad. It is only necessary that in our wish to avoid pain and evil, we do not turn away from the growing edge to which our curiosity leads.'
Sheldon Kopp

A man of 50 came to see me with multiple problems, both at home and at work. He had been in the same job for 30 years and was working below his potential. His wife constantly complained about his inability to make decisions and over the last few years he had developed recurrent incapacitating headaches. He had sought help for these headaches from various doctors and had been told he was suffering from tension. The sedatives he had been prescribed helped ease the pain but made him both lethargic and drowsy.

After many sessions discussing his problem we learnt about his need for the headaches. As a child he had very strict parents who continually complained that he did everything wrong. He didn't dress properly, didn't tidy his room correctly, held his knife and fork wrongly, spoke badly, and so on. As he was growing up, when it was important for him to gain confidence and like himself, all he learnt was that he was good at doing everything incorrectly.

In order to cope with his parents' directions he decided to submerge any initiative of his own and follow their guidance. This at least gave him some measure of peace and a ration of praise and acceptance.

As he grew older and gained responsibilities he found he had minimal experience in decision-making. He became confused, depressed and unhappy and gradually realized that he was left alone whenever he had a headache. At an unconscious level a very useful symptom had developed. It was not unconscious, he was not a malingerer, the head-aches really hurt, but it could be said that he substituted the pain of a headache for the pain of not coping.

The need for a symptom was directly related, via a tortuous and lengthy course, to the removal of a potential during his growing period.

It took a long time and much patience to explore his dormant decision-making ability. It also required consider-able effort by his family and colleagues to support him through his belated growth. However, as he gained con-fidence and took more responsibility, his headaches dimin-ished. They still occurred, but were not so intense and lasted for shorter periods.

Some patients suffering from symptoms of tension, stress and unsatisfactory relationships have an underlying diffi-culty in arguing with their partner. In childhood they grew up with the constant battle of parents screaming at each other and made a definite decision that when they grew up they would never argue. The fear caused by watching or hearing parents fight is so ingrained that such people will do *anything* to avoid an argument; in a relationship they back down every time they sense a disagreement brewing. Their partner often takes advantage of this situation and becomes more demanding or abusive, and over a period of time the confidence of the argument avoider is eroded. The relationship tends to drift apart with one partner trying to hold it together by being subservient and the other partner becoming ever more demanding and discontented. All sorts of symptoms can be associated with the inability to be assertive: tiredness; headaches; obesity; lethargy; all of which may be used to avoid an argument.

These symptoms are a life-raft to be clung to at an unconscious level. The dread of a confrontation is so ingrained that any other inconvenience is preferable. Although attempts to remove the symptoms are repeatedly tried they will remain as long as assertiveness is avoided.

Susan was a mess. Both physically and mentally it was obvious she was not coping well with life. She looked depressed and anxious, her clothes were drab and uncared for, she was grossly overweight and cried constantly. She told a sad story of an unhappy marriage with two children and a rude, overbearing husband. She was apologetic about everything and said 'sorry' constantly. She was sorry she was a minute late, sorry to be a trouble to me, sorry for complaining, sorry almost for being alive. She wanted help for her depressed feeling and constant crying, her weight and sleep problems.

When I commented about her apologizing she said she was sorry for that too. I talked about being more assertive and this brought a new bout of tears. It appeared that her parents constantly fought and she was determined that would never happen in her marriage. She found it so painful to have a confrontation in any area of her life that she became unable to express any opinion differing from her husband's. As time went on he became more aggressive and she became more timid.

No matter how hard I tried I could not encourage her to

stand up for herself. She agreed it might help, but was quite unable to say anything which might result in a row. She ate to comfort herself and to bottle up the feelings she could not express.

After many visits we both realized there was no progress and that I was unable to help her with her many problems. Her early learning pattern was so strong it prevented her living any other way than the one she had chosen with its associated symptoms. She really needed her symptoms as she felt 'she could not cope' without them, even though she was coping very badly with them.

OBESITY AS A SYMPTOM

Obesity is a symptom frequently used as an alternative to dealing with challenges more appropriately. When we were children food was used as a substitute for a multitude of problems. 'Have something to eat, you will feel better' was a phrase constantly repeated as misadventures occurred. As time goes by, life presents its problems and for so many people the habit of 'eating to make it better' has become so ingrained that this is easier than dealing with the problem in a more appropriate and adult way. However, the only problem with using food as a panacea is that it doesn't work. The unfaced situation still exists and the fattened face adds yet another problem.

THE MESSAGE OF SYMPTOMS

In any difficult situation, we have the alternative of making a change in our behaviour or learning to live within our restrictions. Symptoms may appear when the restrictions become too restricting and the limitations too limiting. Or they may appear when, for some reason, we can tolerate the situation no longer. Symptoms help us avoid facing a world we find too difficult to face; a world we 'know' we can't cope with, so we embrace the symptom as the 'only way out'.

However, many, many symptoms are messages to us in the form of comfort, punishment or conflict. Learning to understand them and recognize that they may reflect a situation which is now out-of-date seems an appropriate way to let go of them and grow proportionately.

TURNING POINTS

1 It is possible that the symptom you now have is the best possible choice for the present time.
2 Check if your symptom is helping you avoid something, or if you are gaining in some way from it; what can you learn from it?
3 Ask yourself honestly what benefits and problems you would have without your symptom.
4 Check if you have been receiving suitable help or advice and study alternative areas where help might be more appropriate.

PART 2

Perpetuating the problem

4

Challenging restrictive beliefs

> I believe therefore I can.
> Positive beliefs expand our world while restrictive
> ones shrink it.

My career has changed over the years, like a stream meandering through the meadows. Due to these changes I've gathered titles – doctor, hypnotherapist, counsellor, psychotherapist – so when people asked me what I did for a living it was quite a mouthful. I now reply, 'I challenge restrictive beliefs.'

The basis of this new more succinct title is that most people hold beliefs to steer them through life's challenges. Often these beliefs are out of date, inaccurate and restricting, rather than freeing their life style. Because our attitudes and behaviour are so tightly interwoven with our personality, it is difficult to view our own beliefs from a critical viewpoint. To us they are facts, realities unchangeable.

Mrs Turner was a 50-year-old widow having trouble

coping with her life. She did the best she could but was constantly unhappy, depressed and unable to enjoy life.

Our sessions were spent exploring any fixed beliefs she may have held that were relevant to her problem. She was firmly convinced of the following and related them as facts rather than opinions:

I know I am not a nice person.

I must love *everybody*.

If I try something I'm sure to fail.

Everyone is better (more capable, attractive, etc.) than I am.

If I don't help *everyone* I'll end up in hell.

It was my fault my mother had such an unhappy life.

I know what people think of me.

The list goes on and on, multitudes of sayings she kept repeating to herself closing her life into a shell, husk, preventing any freedom.

My task was to bring those beliefs out into the sunshine of reality and see if they stood the test of being challenged. It was no easy task. She felt very frightened at even discussing these beliefs, let alone discarding them.

We proceeded painfully and slowly for many weeks, slowly teasing out the thoughts and gaining a different perspective on them. After about two months I received a letter cancelling our next appointment and pointing out it was wrong to challenge the structure of her life. Yet another of Mrs Turner's beliefs had put an end to any possibility of achieving freedom.

In order to discover the vast network of attitudes that govern our lives all we need to do is question. I say 'all we need to do' implying it is simple, in fact it is far from simple and requires a 'facilitator' to act as a supportive guide for the process of questioning, doubting challenging to proceed.

The 'questioning' takes the form, 'Why do I do that? What makes me think that? How do I know that belief about myself or others is true? How is it that I have that feeling when I speak my mind?'

These questions lead us to the basic beliefs that run our lives, out of conscious awareness, perhaps since childhood. The cause may be previous experiences, parental indoctrination, misfortunes or painful memories.

As our beliefs guide our lives, it follows that open, freeing, encouraging beliefs will allow us to enjoy our life much more than self-blaming, guilt making or restrictive ones. As I have already said beliefs are not realities yet they influence us as if they are. Our task is to gently tease out the fabrications from the fabric of our personalities and replace them with more appropriate up to date attitudes.

We can change the way we feel by changing the way we look at things even if the situation remains the same.

A friend of mine was distraught and depressed by the behaviour of her teenage son. He was rude, not studying, smoking drugs, staying in bed till midday etc. (Perhaps he could be described as the average teenager.)

She did her best to change this behaviour but all to no avail. Every day brought another crop of tragedies causing her to feel worse.

One day when I met her she was changed. She looked bright and cheerful and I wondered if her son had seen the light. When I asked her if this was so she replied:

'No, he's just the same but I feel so much better because someone has explained it all to me. He is just going through a difficult puberty that is why he is behaving the way he is.'

I stood with my mouth open unable to believe what I was hearing. Here was a mother who had been understandably distraught at her son's most unpleasant behaviour and now she was cheerful because the problem had been reframed as 'a difficult puberty' hence explaining away the problem.

It was then that I realized how powerful changing beliefs can be. The situation at home remained the same, her son misbehaved as he had previously done, but she was smiling and whistling through the day borne aloft by the 'difficult puberty' phrase.

THE MAP IS NOT THE TERRITORY

If we regard our progress through life as being dependent on two factors:

(1) The map used to help us.
(2) The territory we pass through with time.

then we can learn more about our ability to cope.

If the map we use – our beliefs, attitudes – is incorrect, out of date or inappropriate, our journey will be so much more difficult whatever the terrain (experience) is.

Life becomes so much simpler, less stressful, if we have an up-to-date map (suitable and useful beliefs) to help us tackle the problems life tends to put in our way.

LINKING

One specific area of restrictive thinking is formed by 'linking' – connecting two facts with an apparent reason. Life isn't simple and simple explanations are generally brief, easy and wrong.

One hundred years ago antibiotics were discovered. The incidence of disease and mortality improved over the following years. These two facts:

1) Discovery of antibiotics and
2) Improved health

were connected by a 'because':

'The decline in disease occurs because of the discovery and introduction of antibiotics.'

Simple, plausible and wrong.

Historians have shown that the improvement in health at that time was due to improved social conditions – sanitation and sewerage. Nothing at all to do with antibiotics. However the process of linking had occurred by the time the historians reported their findings, and the billion pound pharmaceutical industry was already in place.

Louise is a 50-year-old mother of two. She has great difficulty with life as she has to perform a number of obsessive actions each day such as washing her hands, cleaning the house from top to bottom and making sure everything around her is untainted by germs.

This process takes three hours every day, the rest of the day is spent catching up or exhausted from the compulsive activities.

Her history revealed that she was the only child of parents who fought and argued continuously. One night when she was 7 she was woken by a violent quarrel. She crept downstairs and sat on the staircase watching her parents scream at each other. Her father said he was leaving, her mother replied helplessly that if he left she would kill herself.

In tears Louise crept back to her bed and heard the door slam as her father left in high dudgeon. She was terrified her mother would kill herself and recalled her grandmother saying that if she prayed hard good things would happen.

She got out of bed, knelt down and prayed and prayed that her mother would live. She stayed on the floor for an hour, eventually falling asleep there.

In the morning, in fear and trepidation, she went downstairs and to her joy her mother was still alive.

She made a link. She *knew* her prayers had saved her mother. Every night she prayed beside the bed for an hour to make sure her mother stayed alive. She began to doubt her prayers and devised other methods to keep her mother from dying. As the years passed these actions became more and more time consuming and less rational. She believed washing her hands, being a good clean girl, would help her mother. She continued in this way until the age of 50 – the linking had taken over. She was in the grip of obsessive compulsive actions and was unable to use reason to tackle her plight.

I am not saying all obsessive compulsive disorders originate in this way, as they definitely do not. What I'm saying is that linking is a very powerful, inaccurate and restrictive mechanism we all use without analysing the basis for the connections we accept.

MIND READING

Another false belief threading its way through our lives I call 'mind reading'.

'If I go to the pictures in this dress my boyfriend will think I'm an idiot.'

If I ask a question in class my teacher will think I'm hopeless.'

'If I return those bad apples the greengrocer will get angry.'

How do we have any idea how other people will think? The truth is – we don't and never will. Even if we ask they are unlikely to reply honestly. To be continually concerned about what other people think is a dangerous and destructive game with no basis for confirmation. The sad but real truth is that in most cases PEOPLE DON'T CARE. They are too involved with their own problems to be overly concerned with what you say or how you act. The belief that others are intensely worried about what you say or do is generally false and restricting.

Elizabeth came to see me about headaches troubling her for some months. During the course of our conversation she commented she would love to see a certain film but had no one to go with.

'*Why don't you go on your own?*' I innocently asked.
'Oh I couldn't do that. What would people think?'
'*What people are you talking about?*'
'The other people at the cinema.'
'*I have no idea what they may think. What do you believe they may think and why is it of any consequence?*'

Elizabeth looked at me horrified as if I was talking some indecipherable gibberish.

'You can't be serious Dr Roet. How could I go to the pictures on my own? What would my friends think of me?'
'*I have no idea. Do you know what they would think?*'

'Yes of course, they would be horrified.'

'How do you know that? Have they said as much?'

'No not really but I know that's what they'd think so I can't go.'

I could see I was getting nowhere with logic and as Elizabeth was determined to hold onto her belief I let the conversation drift onto other subjects. Every topic we discussed involved Elizabeth's mind reading ability and the importance of other people's attitudes (or the attitudes she attributed to them).

In fact Elizabeth's life was constricted on all sides by her incorrect beliefs and her headaches were a symptom of this attitude.

When people challenge and disregard their restrictive beliefs they often feel *physically* different as well as happier and more successful.

'I'm actually feeling taller since we discussed the way I look at things.'

'It is as if an actual weight has been lifted. I feel more free, less exhausted.'

'As I listen to other people I now hear how their beliefs create a struggle which is unnecessary.'

TURNING POINTS

1 Spend some time analysing why you do the things you do. What are the underlying beliefs acting as maps for you?

2 Ask yourself if these maps are suitable, helpful and up to date with your needs.

3 Think about some beliefs that are closer to reality (the territory) than the ones you have. Decide on making some changes in this direction.

4 Are you 'linking' two facts together to explain them? Does the linking stand up to logical examination?

5 Are you a 'mind reader'? Are you concerned about what other people think? Is there any way you could test your mind reading? Is it helpful or restrictive?

6 Make a commitment to put some beliefs that are releasing, freeing, into practice, being aware they are still beliefs and not reality.

5

Negative self-talk

'Every day
I think about dying
about disease, starvation, violence, terrorism, war
the end of the world.
It helps
keep my mind off things.'
Roger McGough, *The Survivor*

We all tend to talk to ourselves as a means of keeping in touch with our feelings, hopes, intentions. We may or may not be aware of this continued silent conversation but it is effective just the same. It is as if we are our own chronicler, commentator, coach, judge and jury without being fully aware of the roles we are playing. This self-talk has an extremely powerful influence on how we act or feel – we often react to the words we say to ourselves rather than to the facts as they occur.

Indeed, *telling* ourselves we cannot do something is equivalent to being unable to do it. How many times do we avoid situations, not because of the practicality of the event, but owing to the negative instructions we give

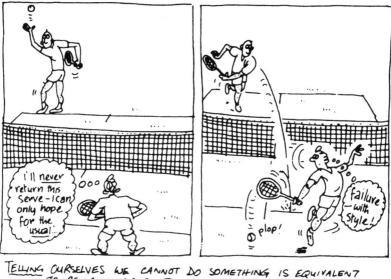

TELLING OURSELVES WE CANNOT DO SOMETHING IS EQUIVALENT
TO BEING UNABLE TO DO IT.

ourselves? A man who has a phobia about lifts tells himself
he cannot go into a lift – and he cannot. Another man finds
the lift locked and is unable to enter it. The internal words
of the first man are as powerful as the lock for the second.
A thousand pounds placed in the lift is out of reach of both
of them.

With a chronic problem, the longer it continues the more
strongly negative the self-talk becomes. If the problem
involves an event which repeats itself (such as sleep
disturbance), a message of failure is transmitted to our
consciousness from the silent babbler in the back of our
mind. The conscious mind obediently follows the instructions so making sure failure occurs and recurs – it is a self-
fulfilling prophecy.

Often the propelling energy of negative self-talk results
from some previous painful, frightening or guilt-making

experience. We keep reminding ourselves of that experience to prevent it recurring. Unfortunately this continued internal warning drains our energy and confidence and a subtle change occurs in the message. Instead of warning ourselves about an earlier calamity, it is as if we are telling ourselves it is likely to happen again in the future. Instead of allowing the past event to drift into the past where it belongs, we continue to carry it with us, reducing our confidence and positive attitude towards similar situations. These continuous warnings from the past create a present-day problem.

Charlie is a very shy man of 25, who desperately wants to meet people, talk to them, and make friends. He is, however, very lonely and painfully shy when in anyone's company. He doesn't speak, looks at the ground, fidgets and blushes. Naturally other people catch his tension and keep away from him.

As a small boy he was quiet and reserved. He was picked on by the bully of the class and the rest of the class joined in the sport of teasing Charlie. He told himself that the best way to avoid the painful experiences he was having was to say nothing at all, then they couldn't pick on him. So he skulked around the school spending all his time avoiding contact with anyone, avoiding saying the wrong thing by keeping silent.

In fact this method didn't help matters much; the other kids still seemed to treat him as the class scapegoat – scribbling in his books, calling him names, playing unkind tricks on him. But he had set a course of action and was unable to change it. As he grew he developed the habit of looking at the ground, avoiding eye contact, pretending not to notice what was going on around him. He was miserable, unable to be positive and spent the school day waiting to get home to the safety of his bedroom.

As he moved from class to class he was no longer picked on and, mistakenly, he believed this was due to his attempted invisibility. The peace of being left alone reinforced his behaviour. He maintained an internal dialogue similar to a soldier in hiding behind enemy lines. His life depended upon him not being seen, not causing any controversy, not being positive.

In his teens he noticed he was in a quandary. He really wanted to make friends, have fun, join in with other boys, but the previous painful experiences warned him about what might happen if he came out of hiding. He told himself he would be laughed at if he gave a differing opinion, and that the old hell would be recreated.

When I saw him he had a job in a library – a suitable place which fulfilled his 'forbidden' speaking role. His shyness was evident by his posture, silence and embarrassment at having to confront a doctor with his long-term secret problem.

Over the course of many sessions we discussed how his negative internal dialogue was out of date. The advice, once suitable for a little boy in class, was no longer appropriate for an adult out of school. We patiently worked at changing the message to one that would allow him to come out of his shell. He needed to improve his social graces, his confidence, his ability to look people in the eye, his speech and conversation. Over many months he gradually experimented to update his internal dialogue.

He began by talking to the bus conductor when he gave his fare; then he spoke to someone in a shop when he bought his lunchtime sandwiches. He commented on the weather or some topical event. We discussed the results of these forays into the real world; sometimes he received pleasant replies, at other times he was ignored.

He had to relearn what he had lost all those years ago. He had to put together piece by painful piece the parts of himself which in fear he had ignored. It was a very slow process but he managed to begin to believe he could voice an opinion and not have all hell break loose as he had anticipated.

CHANGING THE SUBJECT

Negative self-talk may eliminate the possibility of a positive outcome. If you tell yourself you 'can't' do something, this makes it impossible for you to 'try' to do it and so blocks any alternative course of action.

There are not many things you can't do. There are many things that are difficult to do, but if you feel the need you may be able to achieve them. Try to be aware of your internal conversations and whenever the word 'can't' crops up replace it with 'it will be difficult to'. This allows an escape clause in the contract of failure. Notice how you feel when you change 'can't' for 'won't'.

By bringing your mental messages into your consciousness you can become aware of what you are telling yourself. Perhaps the wording is appropriate and can be left as a guide in the unconscious. It is, however, possible that much of what you say is unsuitable for your present objectives and that by assessing and analyzing it you can improve its content.

Often we use negative *riders*; comments on our comments which illustrate our internal negative attitudes. Sayings are commonly heard such as:

'I made dinner for six last night *but I'm such a hopeless cook.*'

'I'm feeling so much better; *but I'm sure it will all go wrong.*'
'I think I did well with what you asked me to do *but I probably made 100 mistakes.*

Our negative self-commands may cause us so much trouble because the mind can only accept positive orders. For example, try not thinking of your nose; immediately your mind focuses *on* your nose in order to know what *not* to think of. In this way, negative self-talk often achieves the opposite of what is intended.

THE CATASTROPHISER

One example of negative self-talk is what I call 'The Catastrophiser'. This person lives in the mind and is often a remnant of one parent or other who constantly proposed doom and gloom.

The tool of the catastrophiser is 'What if ...?'

Whenever a choice occurs and you decide on one course of action, a 'What if ...?' followed by an image of a catastrophe occurs limiting your choice.

Theresa had a very limited life. She was in fear and trepidation of most things that could be considered normal everyday events. Her mother was a very neurotic woman who had constantly reminded Theresa how dangerous the world was.

Theresa's internal dialogue went something like this.

'I think I'll go for a walk in the park this morning.'
Catastrophiser: 'What if you get mugged? You remember the woman last year who nearly died.'

'Oh, that's right. I better not risk it. I think I'll go for a cycle to the shops instead.'

Catastrophiser: 'What if you get a puncture? And anyway the roads are slippery and you may be knocked down by a car.'

'I'm sure I'll be all right. I know I'll ride slowly and very carefully.'

Catastrophiser: 'You're not a good rider. You nearly fell off two years ago. You know you can't trust yourself.'

And so Theresa becomes unhappy, heaves a big sigh and gets on with the boring housework. The catastrophiser goes into hiding with a big smile knowing it has won again. It waits in hiding until another discussion occurs then it comes out with a 'What if?' to start all over again.

The Catastrophiser is a very powerful figure who is not often defeated by logic. It works in the future so it is not possible to be certain it is incorrect. It is like Damacles' sword hanging over our heads. It comes into being by the repeated brainwashing we received in childhood by being told 'Don't do this or that' as terrible things may happen.

It is a worthy opponent as it doesn't give up easily. As soon as you challenge one 'What if?' it is off with another. There is always a lingering sense of doubt that it may be correct and so challenging it is tempting fate. This superstitious thinking is very powerful and resistant to reason.

> 'Out of the gloom, a voice said unto me
> "Smile and be happy, things could get worse".
> So I smiled and was happy, and behold, things
> did get worse.'
> Sign in hospital waiting room

SOME SLIPS OF THE TONGUE

Sometimes the internal self-talk 'escapes' and produces slips of the tongue. These so-called Freudian slips give useful insights into the workings of the mind and are often interesting and humorous.

A woman was married to someone with polio who had a withered arm and leg. There was constant underlying tensions due to his inability to cope with the stresses and strains of life. When I asked her about this she denied it but added, 'When we do have an argument he hasn't got a leg to stand on.'

A female patient came to see me with symptoms relating to guilt and fear. There was some suspicion that she had been molested by her father as a child When I queried this fact she replied, 'Nothing at all happened. If anyone suggests differently it's poppycock.'

A man with sexual problems as a result of a number of difficult relationships was having trouble maintaining an erection. When I asked if he intended starting a long-term relationship in the near future he said, 'I am giving myself a sabbatical from firm commitments for a while.' Another patient with a similar problem commented, 'I'd like to get this thing straightened out once and for all.'

Doctor: 'Are you well in yourself?'
Grossly overweight patient: 'Yes thankyou doctor, by and large.'

A man with a foot deformity who suffered from symptoms of stress and anxiety complained he 'couldn't take things in his stride as he should be able to.'

Many overweight patients comment that the reason they eat is because they are fed up.

A man who had narrowing of his oesophagus (gullet) requiring stretching under an anaesthetic on a regular basis, complained he constantly argued with his wife and she 'always rammed her opinions down my throat!'

An alcoholic when asked about his problem with emotions replied, 'They are all bottled up!'

The above examples illustrate the saying, 'The most important words you will ever hear are those that you tell yourself.'

TURNING POINTS

1 Learn to listen to (and be aware of) your internal language.
2 Note negative self-talk occurring in the form of criticism, doubt or self-fulfilling prophecies.
3 Be aware of words (internal and external) that you frequently use, such as 'can't', 'mustn't', 'shouldn't'.
4 Recognize limitations you are creating by negative commands and alter the wording to a more positive nature.
5 Be aware if a 'catastrophiser' is living in your mind. Notice the 'What ifs?' you are telling yourself and pictures of future catastrophes you are forming in your mind. Challenge the catastrophiser by checking past experience and noting how accurate it has been with its 'What ifs. . .?'

6

Imprinting – the fingerprints of fate

> 'Commands chiselled in the back of the mind,
> weathering the storms of time longer than gravestone
> obituaries and equally as emotional.'

Often we seem to behave according to some previous command or direction. This process has been called imprinting, and if it is of the negative variety may have far-reaching effects for many years after the original incident.

You may think I am talking about some remote brainwashing science fiction scheme but I can assure you I am not. We have all received imprints at some stage in our lives and are carrying them out in some form or another.

An imprint requires three factors:

- a person under stress – frightened, nervous, tense;
- another person of authority with a dominant attitude;
- a command or prediction made by the authoritarian figure.

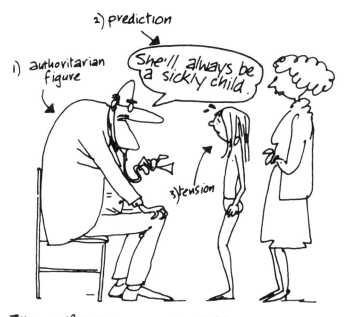

THE INGREDIENTS OF AN IMPRINT

Sometimes the command or statement becomes embedded in the back of the mind as an unquestioned order which *must* be obeyed. This order continues, without the knowledge of the receiver, for years following the initial imprint.

A CROSS SISTER

Tony, who is 32, is terrified of dying. For as long as he can remember he has been afraid of death and in recent years the fear has become worse. He feels he is about to die and dreads the days ahead, knowing it will surely happen soon.

His past history was unremarkable except for two car accidents some years previously – one of them quite serious, the other trivial. His home and working life were normal apart from this constant fear of death that hung over him. He had no idea why he was so frightened of dying and knew how illogical it was, but couldn't shake it off. He was taking sedatives and attending a counsellor to discuss his problems and anxiety. He was not very keen to see me to discuss his problem, feeling it would be of no use to see yet another therapist.

I suggested I might use hypnosis to try to understand how his phobia had developed. I asked him to relax and allow any thoughts to drift into his mind. Over a period of minutes I guided him back to the first time he had felt so strongly about dying. He remained motionless for some minutes then began to talk about a time when as a boy of 10 he had polio and was in hospital. Everyone was very worried about him and from their attitudes he knew he must have been very ill. It was Christmas time and, as his parents were continually visiting the hospital, there was no time to buy presents for his 12-year-old sister.

One day his sister came to his hospital bed and in a very cross, threatening voice told him she wished he was dead so she could get her Christmas presents.

The imprint was formed, the three requirements were present:

- a person under stress – a sick, frightened child in hospital away from home;
- a person of authority – his older sister;
- a statement or command – 'I wish you were dead'.

This imprint had remained dormant until his car accidents when the unconscious mind associated the two incidents as if a spell had been cast.

As he talked to me he said, 'I feel strange, as if I'm getting bigger and bigger' which I took to be a release from his childhood restrictions. Unfortunately the command had had such an effect that he did not make any future appointments, but kept this fear of death and continued to avoid any confrontation with the imprint which had been part of him for so long.

AN EXASPERATED DOCTOR

Doctors are often in a position to inflict negative imprints on their patients; as they have a role of authority they often make powerful statements which may be misinterpreted by frightened patients.

A lady of 60 with a very nervous disposition was frightened of going mad. Her aunt had been in an institution for years and her impressions of visiting her aunt were still vivid. She became depressed for no obvious reason and was put on anti-depressant tablets. Over a period of time her medication was increased to eight tablets a day and two at night. She didn't like taking the tablets as she remembered the nurse handing out tablets to her aunt in the institution. She felt she might be going mad and wanted to stop taking them.

She repeatedly asked her doctor how long it would be necessary to keep taking the tablets. He initially avoided a direct answer but one day he became exasperated by the insistent questioning and snapped at her, 'You'll have to be on the tablets for as long as you live'.

Terrified by this outburst she ruminated for weeks about her condition. She hated taking the tablets but was terrified of reducing them in case she went mad. For four years she remained on 10 tablets a day, dreading the fact that she was 'addicted' to them and determined in some way to stop her dependence on them.

She moved home and went to another doctor who reassured her she was now well and could stop the tablets. But unfortunately, she was caught by the imprint.

'You'll have to be on the tablets as long as you live.'

The new doctor was understanding and sympathetic and gradually reduced the tablets one half at a time. Each time she took one half a tablet less she was unwell for a week. She was tired, had palpitations, became dizzy and retired to bed. She dreaded these confrontations but was determined to get off the tablets.

She came to see me after she had reduced her anti-depressants to three a day and was unable to reduce them any more. Any logic that I put to her about stopping the pills had no effect. Her unconscious mind was terrified at what might happen when she no longer took tablets. The statement 'You must take them as long as you live' seemed to have been interpreted at the back of her mind as 'if you stop you will die'.

I taught her relaxation procedures and discussed at length the psychological aspect of her condition, but she was convinced it was a physical dependence and it would be a big struggle to reduce the tablets any further. And a big struggle it was. We cut the tablets into quarters and every second week reduced them by a quarter. She still had her painful side effects and suffered for some days after each reduction.

Finally, after six months, she was only taking a quarter of a tablet a day and had gained sufficient confidence to go shopping and to the theatre – something she had not done for years. She remained on a quarter a day as a safeguard against the dire prediction of the imprint and we both agreed it would do little harm to remain on a quarter of a tablet a day for many years to come.

We had battled hard against the imprint and respected it

to the extent of not stopping the tablets altogether. She had taken eight years to deal with a situation of depression and an imprint made on the spur of the moment by an irate doctor.

FINDING THE CAUSE

Stern parents or schoolteachers can cause imprints in children, especially when a child is frightened or guilty and the parent or teacher angry. It is as if the words shoot through to the back of the mind and reside there out of reach of the logical, conscious mind, to reappear later as symptoms of a problem which may not even be related to the imprinting incidents, so making change even more difficult.

Even under an anaesthetic imprints can be inflicted on the unconscious patient. It is known that negative statements by surgeons during operations have had far-reaching effects on patients, even though they have no conscious recollection of the event. These statements have been recalled under hypnosis in order to discover the cause of a problem.

Thinking about previous situations where the three components of the imprint were present may enable you to discover what effect, if any, they are having on your life. By looking at your beliefs and behaviour calmly and rationally it is possible to rid yourself of the 'hidden commander' from the past, although it may be difficult to gain access to the imprint, especially if it occurred some years previously. Even then, when you have worked it out, a great deal of understanding and patience will be required to alter its effect.

TURNING POINTS

1   Imprints are commands buried deep in the back of the mind.
2   It is often difficult to recognize if an imprint is affecting your life, and professional help, perhaps hypnosis may be necessary.
3   To become aware if imprinting is causing problems you may recall a situation where the three components were present:
   • you were nervous or frightened;
   • an authority figure such as a parent, doctor or teacher was present;
   • the authority figure made an accusing or commanding statement to you or about you.
4   To bring the imprint to consciousness and remove it, add your present knowledge to the previously remembered situation.
   • Discuss the imprint with a close friend or the person who had caused it.

7

Inner tension – a loss of power

'Bones are not filled with marrow but with black
ingratitude.'
Orthopaedic surgeon, about the failure of fractures
to unite

In our homes, there are sources of energy. We use a heating
system in the winter to ensure we keep warm; whether it is
gas, oil or electricity, it costs money and we instal thermo-
stats and insulation to avoid wasting this energy. Any leaks
in the systems are repaired immediately to prevent loss and
avoid disaster. No-one arriving home to the overpowering
smell of gas would ignore it; dripping taps or leaking water
mains are repaired so that irritation or expense are prevented.

Your body works in a similar way to make energy and
prevent its waste. You sweat to lose heat and shiver to raise
your temperature; you feel tired and the need to rest when
overworked (mentally or physically) and eat when more

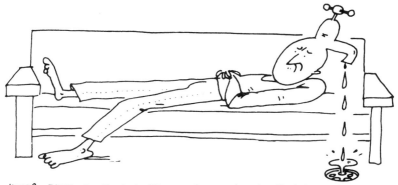

INNER TENSION IS SIMILAR TO RUNNING WATER DRAINING
DOWN A PLUGHOLE ...

power is required; blood vessels seal themselves when cut, and the blood clots to prevent further bleeding.

There is one insidious cause of energy loss which in many cases goes unchecked year after year, and that is the *inner tension*, present to a greater or lesser extent in us all. This inner tension is similar to running water continually draining down the plughole; whether it is a drip or a flood depends on many factors.

The causes of this non-productive waste of energy are many. We know them as anxiety, worry, guilt, conflict, unresolved anger, self-pity, shame and a host of others. All these emotions are using a vast amount of our natural resources for no beneficial result.

Take the common example of a couple who have been married some years and are constantly nagging, fighting and blaming each other for the difficulties in the marriage. You only have to be with such a couple for a few minutes to realize that the continual insults, glares and accusations are as draining as leaving the bathroom tap running for years on end.

In situations such as these the 'fuel' bill is enormous –

dissatisfaction, unhappiness, loneliness, resentment, depression and a host of physical illnesses. If we need our energies to fight off disease (and think of that word as 'dis-ease') it is no wonder that we become ill having wasted that energy in other ways, leaving no reserves to repel external bacteria or viruses.

Eileen was a regular visitor to my surgery. Every two to three weeks she would have a 'genuine' physical illness – severe cold, influenza, headaches, bronchitis, sore throat, ear infection, diarrhoea and so on. Month after month her medical history grew, but when I enquired about her personal life she raised the drawbridge and diverted my questions to her physical ailments.

Only after many months, bottles of antibiotics and days off work did she tell me her underlying problem. After five years of marriage she had discovered her husband was a transvestite. She came home one day unexpectedly from work and found him parading around in one of her dresses. She was understandably distraught and remembered the following weeks as floods of tears, arguments, accusations and utter hopelessness at the situation. Her secret was so painful she could not share it with even her closest friend and lay awake night after night trying to decide what to do. She lost the ability to concentrate at work and kept forgetting even the most simple things. The inner turmoil was burning up her energy like a bonfire.

Whenever she thought about her husband, saw him, met friends with him, the energy bill soared. She stayed up all night with him discussing his problem and how it would affect the family, each of them expressing their feelings – anger, fear, guilt and lack of understanding.

She asked me about seeing someone for counselling and I gave her the name of a suitable therapist who would interview them together and act in a supporting role. After a long time she came to accept the situation and adjust herself to being a more understanding and less blaming partner. As she began to feel better in herself and waste less energy, her physical complaints decreased; she attended the surgery less for pills and more for support. Her body's defences were receiving more of her natural power to combat the bacterial enemies.

THE WORRIER

'I'm just a born worrier, doctor.'

'If I'm not worrying I'm worrying that I'm not worrying.'

'I seem to worry about everyone else's problems as well as my own.'

These are comments from people who came for consultation – drained, depressed and wondering why their lives lacked sparkle and pleasure. It is as if they have a special ability to focus on *any* concern. They create worries where others can find none.

Being concerned, worried, is necessary for survival, but the worrier magnifies this tendency until it becomes destructive. They are ill at ease unless having the comfort of discomfort, that old feeling that is part of them, the niggle that something is wrong. If there are no clouds in the sky they feel different and *know* that they are in for trouble, so they snatch a worry from somewhere.

There are two categories of worry:

1   To worry about things we can do something about.
2   To worry about things we can do nothing about.

It is most important to divide worries into these two categories and put energy into the first – and do something, leaving the second as 'a nuisance to be accepted' not 'a problem to be solved'.

Worriers are a strange breed. They often steal other people's problems rather than letting them sort things out for themselves and grow from the experience. Generally they learn their trade from over-protective parents who are continually giving the message that the world is a dangerous place. As they grow up a belief is developed: 'If I worry it will prevent catastrophes from occurring.' This is a form of magical thinking and it is not easy to discourage. I suggest to worriers that they start a 'worry diary'. This is an exercise book where worries are noted down and divided into the two categories. In the same book an assessment of how inaccurate the worries have been may well diminish their hold.

It is very difficult to discuss facts with a worrier on a logical level as responses such as:

'I can't help it'.
'I've been like this all my life how can I change now?'
'It's a part of me, I'm frightened to let go of it.'

At the same level there are benefits to the worrier in spite of their repeated expressions of desire to be rid of the affliction. Support, attentive listening and concern are often the ingredients required to create change. Confidence is built up to help the person learn that they (and everyone else) will survive without the supposed security of excessive worry.

Question:
'How do you make God laugh?'
Answer:
'Tell Him your future plans!'

DANGER – TENSE MUSCLES

How do we know if our energy is being continuously drained? The body has many warning systems but we may need to be trained to be alert to them. Muscle tension is one such warning device: clenched fists, stiff necks, headaches, clenched jaws, worried frowns and stiff posture are all signs of muscular tension and may mean that electrical impulses are causing muscles to contract unnecessarily. However, once you are aware of this and your muscles' state of tension, you can use them as a barometer measure to internal pressure.

Another group of muscles are outside our conscious awareness; these muscles occur in blood vessels and internal organs such as glands, bowel or bladder. Problems arise if they are continually bombarded with wasteful energy, for example, high blood pressure or heart problems and bowel disorders such as diarrhoea or constipation. This wasted energy is not only lost but causes harmful physical conditions. Again we can use these conditions as an indication that all is not well and that inwardly we are tense.

Becoming aware of the side effects of this energy loss allows us to slow down the flow and reduce the harmful side effects. This awareness may be brought about by diagnostic methods such as checking the blood pressure, bowel X-rays or cardiographs or by learning more about our bodies and how they are indicating internal stress.

LOSING ENERGY

Mental attitudes play a major role in both the loss of energy and the blocking of access to it. People who constantly worry, are nervous, frightened, resentful or guilty, cause symptoms due to the wastage of vital power: lethargy, immobility, exhaustion, pessimism, tiredness, lack of interest, inability to concentrate, poor memory, failure to make decisions, depression, all indicate a breakdown in the essential 'fuel supply'.

Lorraine likes playing tennis; she is a very good player and always arrives on time enthusiastic and vivacious; her bright chatter and laughter always lift the tone of the game irrespective of the scores. Recently she arrived late, shoulders slumped, not smiling and proceeded to play very badly in silence. She was unable to keep the score and showed no enthusiasm as the game proceeded. The explanation came later when she related how she had encountered many difficulties during the previous few days in her new job; the final straw came when her washing machine broke down and flooded just as she was setting off for tennis.

Lorraine's energy was being drained in a similar manner to the water flooding her kitchen floor; her reserve was depleted and none was left for her game of tennis. The incident illustrates just how easily we can fail to be in the 'here and now' because our attention and energy is focused on the past or future. Lorraine's worries about her new job and old machine had no useful effect on either situation, but merely siphoned off any power necessary to play and enjoy the tennis.

People who are depressed display this depletion of vitality to a marked degree. Just as a car running out of fuel can only chug along, barely making the distance, so a depressed person is often like one of those mechanical toys whose battery has run down. Their face is expressionless, movement minimal and slow, voice low and negative, they sleep poorly, have no interest or enthusiasm and are understandably pessimistic about most things. It is often difficult to stem the outflow of energy and regain lost power. A host of possibilities are available from a variety of therapies ranging from tablets to aromatherapy, but as the person suffering the loss has no enthusiasm (like a car without a starter motor) encouraging them to improve their motivation is often time-consuming and frustrating.

A person living in a house with an unrepaired gas leak is irresponsible, and so is the person allowing inner tension to drain their energy. People learning to understand themselves, their problems and how stress is playing a major role, make remarks such as, 'I'm feeling so much better, less tired, more optimistic, I notice things I didn't know existed' and so on, all indicating the 'power supply' is producing a brighter picture.

Keeping emotions 'under control' is often a waste of energy. Not accepting a feeling and 'keeping the lid on it' requires a lot of power. As time goes by and more ingredients are added to the pressure cooker, more energy is required to keep the lid on. Learning to feel free to accept and express emotions releases this power, enabling it to be used in other directions (see page 160).

Spending time and effort to check your system for leaks may be a very worthwhile exercise for the journey ahead. Not many of us would travel on a long car journey without checking the oil, petrol, water and tyres; a similar internal check-up on yourself will prove a very valuable insurance policy.

Another major cause of energy loss is the type of conflict already mentioned that occurs in the back of your mind, when part of you would *like* to do one thing, but the other part feels you *should* do something else. The tug of war that continues outside your conscious awareness drains power and gets you nowhere. Understanding and resolving the conflict releases energy for more fruitful purposes.

There are many ways of diminishing internal strain; learning to slow down, having time to relax, doing meditation or self-hypnosis, having a regular massage. Gaining an understanding of the external and internal conflicts continually at play will enable you to direct attention to the trouble spots.

Most people start with the best intentions but soon lose interest and enthusiasm; their half hour a day soon becomes 10 minutes, then 'I'll do it later' and eventually forgotten until the symptom rears its ugly head again.

Both the cause and solution are within your control, and the decision to put them into practice rests with you alone.

TURNING POINTS

1 Inner tension is a cause of long-term symptoms and drains energy.

2 Learn to recognize signs of internal tension such as clenched fists, tight muscles, grinding teeth, hunched shoulders.

3 Check whether your symptoms, high blood pressure, bowel problems, headaches, are a result of tension.

4 Take steps to stop the loss of energy, diminish the tension by relaxation, meditation, massage, self-hypnosis.

5 Understand the mechanism producing the internal conflict and take steps to deal with the external factors.

8

The sinister partners of fear and guilt

'In everyone there sleeps
A sense of life lived according to love.
To some it means the difference they could make
By loving others, but across most it sweeps
As all they might have done had they been loved.'
Philip Larkin, *Faith Healing*

'For every action that is not expressed because of fear, for every desire that wells up in the breast and is not given vent in action through fear turns into a little rat of guilt that gnaws away at your vitals.'
Steven Berkoff, writing on Kafka's book *The Trial*

In order to understand why a situation continues, in spite of repeated comments indicating a desire for the reverse, it is worthwhile analyzing the factors which aid the perpetual motion of the long-term problem.

A multitude of apparently unrelated factors provide the

energy to maintain the unwanted problem, and without discovering and dealing with them, the problem often cannot be resolved. The oiling of the machinery is provided by emotions, attitudes and opinions, the most common of which are fear and guilt.

FEAR

In any given situation where alternatives are available, a frightened person will inevitably anticipate the worst – the most fearful and negative choice. It is possible that this is a survival mechanism, inherited from primitive man. If a caveman on hearing a noise, assumed it was a friend dropping in for a meal, he might have been devoured by a sabre-toothed tiger. On the other hand, if he was prepared for the worst, he would survive.

A frightened person alone in a house at night will interpret a moving curtain as a burglar, while during the day, in daylight and with people passing on the street, the same person would have realized that it was just the wind blowing the curtain.

Anyone with a long-term underlying fear, for whatever cause, will be pessimistic about any positive outcome to the problem and will be extremely sensitive to any negative word or voice tone and anticipate the worst possible outcome.

A woman I saw recently, constantly anxious about her health, had been to her doctor three weeks before her visit to me. He had given her a thorough check-up and then patted her on the back saying, 'You are pretty fit Mrs Smith'.

She left his surgery in a daze. The words 'pretty fit' somehow conveyed to her that all was *not* well. 'Why didn't he say I was 100 per cent fit? I thought I detected a worried tone in his voice. I'm sure there is something wrong and he didn't tell me because he knew it would make me nervous.'

She continued this train of thought, feeling worse as each day went by. Her underlying fears had directed her to notice things that were not there. She was too frightened to ring and ask the doctor if all was well. Her anxiety caused her to lose her appetite which reinforced her beliefs.

When she saw me she was a 'bundle of nerves' and needed constant reassurance that all was well. I 'phoned her doctor in her presence and he too explained she was completely fit. She left, still unconvinced but on the road to letting go of her anxiety. I felt, however, that it would not be long before she would misinterpret something else and start the process of worrying again.

As with imprinting (see page 67), the initial fear underlying a long-term problem may result from a situation that occurred several years previously, perhaps in childhood. It is as if the person has been 'sensitized' by one or more frightening experiences and so is 'on guard' against any future calamities. Although the original fear may be forgotten and far removed from the present chronic condition, it nevertheless erodes any possibility of a solution.

Dealing with the fear is a major step in the right direction and this is done by first realizing that it exists. Many people with underlying fears do not interpret their uncomfortable feelings correctly. By examining bodily sensations and associated thoughts we can learn if fear is playing a role in maintaining our problem. These sensations may vary from tight jaw muscles, a 'hollow feeling' in the pit of the stomach, being 'on edge', to a full blown panic attack – racing pulse, rapid breathing and 'terror' in the eyes.

Underlying fear is also often expressed as resistance to change; any suggestion is met with negative comments. It is as if the fear of something worse occurring provides a reason for maintaining the *status quo*, however uncomfortable that may be, as in the case of Susan (see page 44).

Jacqueline's case is rather similar, although it has a happier outcome. She is a 35-year-old secretary and when she first came to see me she was 18 stone and had been that weight for five years. She had tried numerous ways of losing weight, all only temporarily successful. After some discussion I asked her what benefit she had in staying fat. She replied there was no benefit, it was a nuisance, she couldn't get any clothes to fit and so on. I repeated the question and asked her to think about it and let any thoughts or words come from the back of her mind.

After a minute or so she said, 'Because it's safer being fat', and then looked amazed that she could utter such strange words. 'What do you mean by being safer?' I queried.

'I have no idea, the words just seemed to come out without me thinking.'

'Perhaps somewhere at the back of your mind you associate being thin with being unsafe or threatened.'

'I've never been happy when I was thin. I had so many problems with my ex-husband and other men. Since I've put on all this weight I feel much happier in myself although upset by the weight.'

It turned out that Jacqueline had experienced immense problems relating to men until she put on weight. Since then she had made many good friends with gay men and no longer felt threatened. At the back of her mind she associated the happiness directly with her increased weight and was frightened that if she lost weight she would become thin and unhappy as she had been previously.

She spent some time each day analyzing the fear and realizing that the situation had changed since she was 'thin and unhappy' and that her present happiness was related to a multitude of factors, not solely to being fat. As she accepted the fact that it was not frightening to be thin, she began to lose weight and at the same time reassure the back of her mind it was all right to do so.

Removing or understanding underlying fear is like taking off the brake while travelling in the car. It allows natural optimism and positive attitudes to come into play.

Probability versus possibility In our daily lives we base our actions on the *probability* of events occurring with the knowledge that there is a remote *possibility* of negative situations arising. We take these negative possibilities into account but don't let them dictate our lives. Walking down the street we are aware of the remote possibility of a slate falling off a roof but we don't remain indoors or put on a crash helmet before going out. The probability is that all will be well so we follow that belief.

Someone with underlying fear often pushes negative possibilities into the probability category and acts as if they are a probability.

Joanna has a fear of being bitten by a fish. This was no ordinary fear of fish, for not only would she not swim in the sea, she would not swim in a pool in case a fish had got in there by mistake. Her well-meaning sister suggested they should buy a tropical aquarium so that Joanna would become accustomed to fish and feel comfortable with them. Joanna flatly refused even to consider the suggestion. Her reason for not giving it a try was 'What if a fish gets out of the tank and bites me?' I had to laugh at the picture she created of a tiny fish snapping at her as she ran around the room.

We can understand Joanna on the basis that her underlying fear is so great that any logic is completely overlooked. Her original fear may have been far removed from fish, but the possibility of danger had been pushed so far into the probability compartment of her mind that even the most far-fetched and ridiculous possibility assumed the proportions of a probability.

FEAR OF CHANGE

Perhaps the most powerful aspect of fear is *a fear of change*. This may be a basic component of nature applied to all life forms – from insects to man. Change of situation creates a resistance and energy is used to maintain the status quo.

When people come to see me for change they bring with them a part that is frightened to change. The motto of this part is: 'Better the Devil you know than the one you don't.'

The fear of change needs to be overcome to ensure a successful outcome of therapy. It is a very powerful influence and projects doom and gloom at every opportunity. It points out things aren't all that bad and the techniques used are unlikely to work.

The conqueror of the fear of change is *'risk taking.'* By taking small risks we enlarge our world, providing learning from experience. The conflict between remaining as you are or changing is underneath every thought, action and emotion during therapy. As one patient, who was anxious for a year, stated: 'The thought of change terrifies me, but I just can't bear remaining as I am.'

Fearing fear Often the underlying fear is not directed at any particular situation and may re-energize itself as the *fear of fear*. The sufferer becomes frightened of being frightened and this produces the perpetual motion that recurs in long-term problems. It is as if part of the mind has been programmed 'be on guard at all times and you will be protected'. Unfortunately this is not sound advice as being on guard drains energy creating fatigue, anguish and despair. A nightwatchman who jumps up every time a leaf moves will be far from his peak if real trouble occurs.

Continuous underlying fear immobilizes people or guides them in a downward spiral. In time they become extremely sensitive to any negative input. They find disasters everywhere, notice aches and pains, blemishes, minute alterations in weight and so on. The 'negative detecting mechanism' is sensitized to such a degree that all pessimistic information is greatly magnified. Such people have become prisoners of fear. To any onlooker their prison doors are open or non-existent, but to themselves they are tightly locked by the fear of fear. Encouragement to be more relaxed, to change, to have a different attitude is met with strong resistance; they 'know' they cannot escape, are not free like others around them.

The present situation may be unpleasant but the fear of changing it is worse. Fear is the jailer, smiling, jangling his keys and pointing to the open door, secure in the knowledge they will not leave.

Confronting and solving problems is often a painful process which most of us attempt to avoid; this very avoidance results in greater pain and an inability to grow.

'To those seeking change a great deal of courage is required, comparable to that of a soldier going into battle. They may even be regarded as more courageous than the

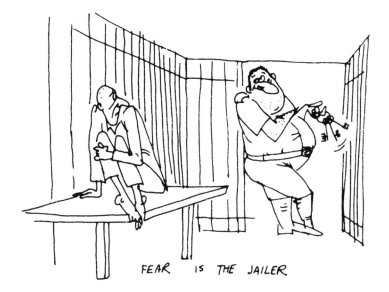

FEAR IS THE JAILER

soldier, by confronting risks more personal and therefore more fearsome and frightening. The soldier cannot run because the gun is pointed at his back as well as his front. The individual trying to grow can always retreat into the easy and familiar patterns of a more limited past.'
M. Scott Peck, *The Road Less Travelled*

GUILT

'True guilt is guilt at the obligation one owes to oneself to be oneself.'
R.D. Laing, *Self and Others*

Guilt is another emotion, often associated with fear, which provides energy for the merry-go-round. It is a very powerful emotion, as we all know having experienced it many times in our lives. Parents often use guilt to make us behave according to *their* standards. 'You shouldn't do that', 'Don't you know it is wrong to behave like that?', 'Fancy a nice boy like you saying a terrible thing like that', 'Don't play with that thing or you'll go blind'.

The classic joke about guilt describes a Jewish mother who gives her son two ties for his birthday. When he next sees her, he is wearing one of his new ties. Her first comment is 'What! You don't like the other tie!'

The constant criticism and belittling of our own beliefs, actions and sayings destroys our confidence in ourselves and we distort ourselves to fit into the uncomfortable requirements of the self-appointed critic. Soon we take over the role of self-critic and force ourselves to live by someone else's standards.

Feeling guilty implies that we are not living up to those standards, however long ago they were set or irrelevant they may be now. This feeling prevents us from acting according to our own beliefs. Guilt is dealt with by punishment. By feeling guilty we unconsciously create self-punishment, and until the guilt is removed it is very difficult to let go of the symptoms acting as self-punishment. Guilt leads to a loss of self-confidence; it seems to be the soil in which weeds grow, crowding the garden and preventing healthy plants from flourishing.

Recognizing the enemy How do we recognize when unconscious guilt is present? Messages from the back of the mind are often interpreted by actions or words. If underlying guilt is present it shows itself in such phrases as: 'I must admit ...', 'I feel guilty about ...', ' I shouldn't do that ...', 'I feel bad about ...', 'I must confess ...'.

Further questioning may uncover guilty feelings not previously discussed or recognized; analyzing feelings the body is experiencing in relation to these attitudes often helps the discovery of the underlying guilt. People often limit themselves – their thoughts, actions, feelings – out of a sense of guilt, although they may not realize that this is the restricting force.

Of the many emotions we have, guilt seems to be the least beneficial. Anger, fear, happiness, sadness all have a useful place in our armament against the world, guilt manipulates us with no benefit to ourselves. It is a stultifying, eroding emotion, draining our self-esteem and confidence. It is as if we are playing a game by someone else's rules; the world asks us to play tennis but we are not allowed to use our forehand.

Guilt has been rather aptly described as 'the difference between what your spirit sings out for and what (action) your courage permits you to take'. Think about this and look out for the ways in which guilt is limiting your beliefs, your feelings and your strengths. Guilt could be turning you into a constant loser, and this too fits the picture, as there is the benefit of self-punishment for failure.

Ursula, a friend of mine who had been fighting depression for a long time, and was coming out of the darkness into the light, wrote me the following note after a particularly courageous effort to overcome her self-criticism:

> I gave my blamer a holiday and said if he found someone else to blame – stay with them! I then asked my praiser to come for tea, and said, 'I'm a bit bored with praising myself, for a change come and praise me'. When he arrived he was surprised to find me alone.
>
> 'Where is your friend, the one who is always with you? I forget his name?'
>
> 'Oh, he has gone, his name was Blamer; I found him so oppressive he wouldn't let me be; nothing I did was

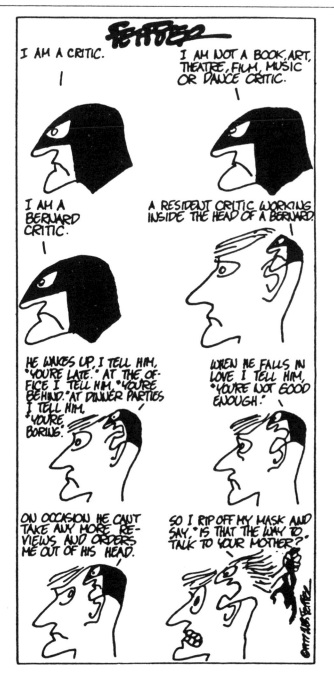

ever right, I'm glad he's out of my sight.'

'Now that you mention it I'm sure you were right,' my lovely praiser said. 'I never liked that fellow, congratulations, because of your foresight and courage you're no longer a child.'

And I smiled and I smiled and I smiled.

The seeds of this treadmill of guilt are often sown early in life when our individuality was not recognized or allowed to develop. So, observing juvenile experiences from an adult point of view may allow us to minimize or remove the unnecessary guilt that has been dogging our heels for years. By following the 'guilt trail' we are often led back to childhood.

A 50-year-old woman obsessed by fear and guilt since her sadistic parents continually blamed her for every thought and deed, commented that she was incapacitated by her feelings. During an interview she remarked, 'The only thing I am good for is to be punished and cry. I am not allowed to be happy because then I'll be punished more; I know worse things are around the corner when I'm happy, and I get very frightened.'

You may now begin to realize the power guilt has in maintaining the merry-go-round of long-term suffering. Unless you can shake it off you are caught at every turn and encouraged to carry on with the suffering circle of guilt – failure – punishment. As time goes on it becomes such a part of life you barely know it exists, in fact you feel guilty if you don't feel guilty.

> 'Can man's mind be his own enemy?'
> 'Mine never gives me any peace.'
> From *Yol*, a film by Yilmaz Guney

TURNING POINTS

1   Underlying fear will cause you to choose the most negative option available when presented with alternative choices.

2   Fear causes negative possiblities to become probabilities and decides decisions accordingly.

3   Fear in the back of the mind is often misdirected to a present-day situation instead of the past experience where it originated.

4   Analyzing the feelings associated with fear may allow its release and replacement with more appropriate attitudes.

5   When fear creeps in logic rushes out.

6   Many people are incapacitated by fear of failure, others by fear of success; each is equally immobilizing.

7   Guilt requires punishment as its rightful due. Often out-of-date and trivial 'crimes' receive life-time sentences.

8   Becoming aware that you are carrying a guilty feeling and 're-trying' the case with up-to-date evidence may allow a 'reprieve'.

9   Counselling, psychotherapy or hypnosis may be required to bring to light the unconscious fear and guilt maintaining chronic symptoms.

10 Look back at episodes in your life when you did or said something which could be responsible for prolonged guilt. Analyze those situations from a present-day point of view.

11 'Facing up' to internal guilt and fear is the best way they can be removed. In the majority of cases the 'confrontation' is much less uncomfortable than expected.

9

Mad, bad or misunderstood

'No-one can make you feel inferior without your consent.'
Eleanor Roosevelt

In relationships, differences of opinion can either be accepted by each partner, fester as unresolved conflicts or be used to label one person mad or bad, thus forcing the relationship apart.

This labelling may be overt, by accusation, or covert, by inference or innuendo. The looks, sneers and comments are many and varied, but all have a similar implication – that the action or statement was that of someone not in their right mind or else who was otherwise malicious; no-one else would do such a thing.

This attitude is generally incorrect and plays no role in resolving any conflict; instead it adds fuel to a smouldering fire. In every relationship there are many differences of attitude, belief, moral standards and behaviour so it is understandable that conflicts of opinion and misunderstandings will occur. When they do, one of two stances may be taken:

- I'm right therefore you are wrong;
- you and I are different.

As you can imagine, when someone has the first attitude it is not a major step for the label mad or bad to become firmly attached to the other partner for holding the views they express.

On the other hand, by taking the second course and agreeing to have differences and accepting those differences, it becomes possible to understand and perhaps learn from the other's experiences.

In long-term relationship difficulties, one major factor in maintaining problems is the view that the other partner is wrong (therefore mad or bad) and so not worthy of respect.

'You forgot to pick up the kids from school, what's wrong with you?'

'You must be mad to think I'd go to dinner with the Joneses after what happened last time.'

'Can't you even budget for two weeks at a time without getting us into debt?'

'How stupid can you be to leave the top off the toothpaste.'

All these accusations, whether made in the heat of the moment or calculated, have the underlying implication that the opposite person fits into the mad or bad category. We all know how such people should be treated, by the psychiatrist or the police, so it does not bode well for an amiable or equal resolution to the continuous inherent difficulties that arise. The mad or bad label wields the powerful club of guilt (see page 89) and great strength is required on the part of the accused to avoid being brow-beaten into submission.

In time the label sticks and the mad or bad one believes that is what he or she is. They are in the wrong and so must pay for the terrible behaviour they are exhibiting in order to break free of the collar of guilt. There are so many opportunities to use this label in any relationship that, if it is accepted, the game of prosecutor and defendant becomes a major part of domestic life.

In childhood being made to feel guilty is a powerful weapon of parental control. Children are regularly subjected to moralizing attacks by their parents:

'Eat up your dinner like a good boy' – inferring that you are bad if you don't.

'Your sister Annie is a good girl, she doesn't do things like that' – Annie is good, you are bad.

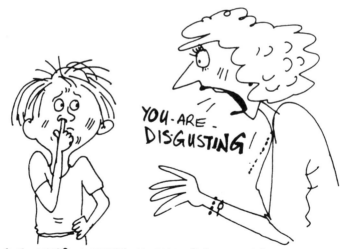

ONE MAJOR MISTAKE IS THAT PARENTS LABEL
THE CHILDREN RATHER THAN THE ACTION ...

'What a foolish child you are spilling your milk like that.'

As children are dependent and need love they will respond to any accusation of badness or madness by trying to please.

A major mistake that parents make is to label the *child* rather than the *action*. If the action is unsuitable it is possible to leave the child's character uncriticized and comment on the deed. In the heat of the moment, however, the child and the action are often fused together by the accusation. Whenever this situation is repeated a tape in the back of the mind runs, saying, 'I'm no good, therefore, I cannot assert myself, succeed or be liked', so laying the foundations for dangerous negative self-esteem.

Very few people say or do things because they are mad or bad. We do things because our abilities and beliefs direct us to and although these differ between people they generally conform to our own moral standards.

As we grow the 'mad or bad' image is ingested and we really come to believe it. This in itself creates problems of low self-esteem, guilt and lack of confidence.

Another problem is caused by this self-depreciating belief. We all have a need to be loved. The person who believes he is bad has an even greater need to be loved but at the same time rejects it on the basis he is unlovable.

An intense and painful conflict is created. It is similar to a plant dying of thirst but coating its leaves with water-proof material to repel the rain.

The need for love, support and understanding is crucial, but when offered it is rejected. A protective cover encircles him so no one will discover his terrible secret – how bad he is inside. Relationships are kept at a safe distance and a variety of defence mechanisms used for survival.

At the same time as this defence battle is being fought a terrible emptiness, sadness and negative attitude dwells within. The process of seeking and rejecting continues from relationship to relationship with despair, helplessness and hopelessness being the result.

The mistakes and failures that do occur can be explained in many different ways; understanding those reasons and appreciating the causes and limitations will go a long way towards removing the momentum of accusations and inferences which cause so much damage. It may be difficult to discuss openly and honestly how mistakes and misunderstandings have occurred, but it is a pathway which leads in a positive direction. As we all have such different ways of doing things it is unlikely there is one way which is correct.

Finding alternative ways to the mad or bad labelling means slowing down the merry-go-round of repeated accusations and guilt, allowing a more positive pathway to be built to the future.

TURNING POINTS

1 In any relationship there will be different points of view, values or ways of doing things. Putting yourself in the other person's position may enable you to appreciate and accept their attitudes.

2 Check how often you use criticism as a means of expressing a difference.

3 Differentiate between the 'action' and the 'person' when commenting on a situation that differs from your belief.

4 Note how many times you assume a moralizing attitude towards your partner or child and observe its effect.

5 Be aware (and beware) of the 'mad or bad' vocabulary you may use in discussions.

10

The doctor's role

'Physicians would rather see a patient die according to the
rules, than recover in an unorthodox manner.'
Molière

'Nobody needs unnecessary operations; and excessive use
of drugs can create dependence or allergic reactions,
or merely enrich the nation's urine.'
Melvyn Werbach, *Third Line Medicine*

As we have discussed already, doctors can cause negative
imprints (see pages 70–71). They are also often involved in
maintaining long-term problems. However, if you are
aware of how doctors are trained, and the attitudes this
training inevitably instils, you may be able to avoid getting
caught in this trap.

Doctors, like myself, receive six or more years' training.
We are taught about the body in all its aspects – anatomy,
biochemistry, pathology and physiology. Detailed analysis
of the intricate parts and workings of the body are studied.
Student doctors are tested on their knowledge of the body,

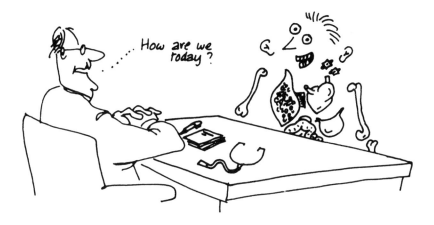

... How are we today?

A DOCTOR'S TRAINING CAN LEAVE HIM LIMITED IN HIS UNDERSTANDING OF THE PATIENT AS A WHOLE.

both in health and illness, until they pass their final exams, their minds crammed with knowledge.

In all those years only a few days are spent learning about the mind. Some lectures about psychiatrically-disturbed people and perhaps a visit to a mental hospital complete the learning about the abnormal mind, even though it is generally acknowledged that a great many of the patients that a doctor will meet in general practice require help with emotional problems. The mind plays a major role in either causing or maintaining chronic illness, but doctors are often ill-equipped to deal with these situations. Our training was not concerned with the fears and worries of the patients; we were mainly interested in finding the diseased organ so we could pass our exams.

Although, with experience, many doctors come to realize the increased tension and anxiety caused by long-term illnesses, they are often wary, or unaware of the methods of relaxation which might help their patients. In our training, drugs and operations were the principal forms of treatment; disciplines such as meditation, yoga, acupuncture or hypnosis were not discussed at all.

As patients most of us go to the doctor when we have a symptom – something for the doctor to 'fix'. This may be useful for acute (short-term) conditions but is not the right approach for chronic (long-term) conditions. It is very difficult indeed to 'fix' many long-term problems with tablets or operations. Of course there are some conditions which require and respond to corrective operations, such as hip replacements and the removal of cataracts, but many of the conditions crowding outpatient clinics and doctors' waiting rooms do not respond to the 'fixing' attitude.

The problem of the long-term patient belongs to the long-term patient, who must accept responsibility for the difficulty. The role of the doctor, in my opinion, is really to act as guide, adviser, supporter, teacher and someone who understands the situation and offers alternative points of view, encouraging the patient to use his or her own resources.

If the doctor is given the patient's problem to 'fix', there are often repeated attempts and failures which only add to the difficulties. If the doctor accepts this role in the mistaken belief that tablets and tests will fix the problem, the chances are that the doctor will become as frustrated and disappointed as the patient. A false contract is being agreed upon which will not result in satisfaction for either party.

Time is also a major factor in being of help to the whole person. The quickest way to see a patient is to give a prescription, but this can compound the initial difficulties presented to the doctor. Medication may have side-effects or a habit-forming quality, so that if the symptoms are temporarily relieved they will recur when the medication is

stopped. In order to extricate themselves from the quicksand, doctors prescribe more powerful drugs and more
tests.

*The most expensive piece of equipment ever produced is
the ballpoint pen. Doctors can write a thousand pounds'
worth of tests and treatment in ten minutes.*

If the psychological component of the condition is
ignored and all the efforts of patient and doctor are
concentrated on the 'symptom', the merry-go-round continues. Many times the symptom is just a guide to be
followed to the real difficulties which lie in the mind.
Medical training to examine, analyze, test and treat the
symptoms of an illness is vital to help the body rid itself of
acute diseases. In chronic conditions recognition of the
mind's role is essential if any progress towards solving the
problem is to be made.

The British Holistic Medical Association has for its
motto, 'Physician Heal Thyself'. To be of the greatest help
to the public, it is important that we feel at peace with
ourselves. The unrest doctors feel due to their own circumstances is easily transferred to the patient. There is much
controversy about alternative or complementary medicine
and where it fits in with orthodox medicine. I feel the
division would be more suitable if it was between good and
bad doctors. The former have an open mind both to their
patients and to alternative forms of therapy available. The
latter have fixed, inflexible ideas, are not open to suggestions advocating different therapies and so limit the benefits available to their patients.

TURNING POINTS

1   The doctor is the mainstay of help in disease but
    the patient must take responsibility for his or her
    chronic illness.
2   A little knowledge may be a dangerous thing, but
    understanding what is wrong with you and asking
    questions about your problem is your right and
    privilege.
3   Alternative or complementary forms of medicine
    may well be of help in addition to the orthodox
    doctor.
4   If the doctor does not have time to listen and
    prescribes tablets instead, it may be worthwhile
    seeking someone else to answer your questions
    or acknowledge your beliefs.
5   Chronic conditions have psychological compo-
    nents as well as physical ones and both need help.

PART 3

Understanding ourselves

11

The importance of understanding

'Being understood is similar to being loved.'
Long-term pain patient

The more you learn to understand yourself – and your problem as part of yourself – the better able you will be to deal with it. It is also true that if you do not understand yourself, you will not be able to understand, and help, others.

Some interesting aspects of understanding others may be related to how we see ourselves. Often we never think about ourselves and spend minimal time in accepting or understanding our beliefs or attitudes. One therapist asked each patient to look in a mirror for 30 seconds. There was a wide variety of results ranging from tears to fear. One patient threw the mirror against the wall and left the room. If we are unable to look at ourselves for 30 seconds it is hardly likely that we can understand ourselves.

When we have symptoms – pain, irritation, sleeplessness – we often *blame* the part responsible or ourselves for allowing it to occur. I have found on many occasions that if the patient changes their attitude to the part causing trouble and tries to *understand* it, rather than blame it, things improve.

Cyril had had headaches for months. He was studying very hard for an exam and became extremely annoyed that the headaches were interfering with his work. I asked him about his attitude to these persistent headaches.

'They are a bloody nuisance', he replied. 'If I fail because of them I'll be really angry. I want to work hard but I can't do my best with these persistent headaches.'

I suggested to him that perhaps the headaches were a result of all the tension and might even be a message to him to slow down a little. I suggested that if he altered his attitude towards his headaches he might find some improvement. I guided him to *understand* his pain rather than *blame* it.

Over the next few weeks the pains subsided considerably as if the head was responding to being accepted and understood and no longer needed to cause pain.

Understanding yourself, however, is not everything. *Being understood* is vitally important to people with chronic long-term problems.

'Sometimes just being alive feels like having no skin, just raw flesh . . . vulnerable, responsive, irritable, in constant danger. Those are the times when I need most to sense my place among other people, to hear their tale and know that it is mine as well. I need so badly to be sure that someone can hear me, to receive his answering cry, to respond in kind.'

Sheldon Kopp, *The Hanged Man*

In any situation, whether between two adults in love, a child/parent or child/teacher relationship or between doctor and patient, one of the most important requirements for the resolution of a difficulty is *being understood*. It may sound simple and common sense but often in communication one person's comments are completely misinterpreted.

This was exemplified by a pain group I was involved with in a London hospital. Eight people suffering from long-term pain met each week for an hour or two to discuss their problems. The sites of pain varied from person to person, but the unifying aspect that they were all chronic sufferers allowed them to speak with understanding. All the participants had received extensive investigation and treatment in the form of tablets, operations, acupuncture or physiotherapy. The causes of their pain were varied and they all maintained little benefit had been gained from previous treatment.

We talked about many different aspects of their lives and found they had one major complaint about society – *not being understood properly*. Each in turn expressed in their own way how they felt misunderstood by their doctors, friends and relatives – having no visible sign of their disease they failed to receive the sympathy and understanding they required. They were all sensitively programmed to notice the negative responses received when talking about their complaints.

After two sessions everyone unanimously agreed that the benefit of the group was in being understood. As they were all in 'the same boat' they felt a kinship they had not previously experienced. They also felt freer, less guilty, less restricted, more acceptable, and this energy was helpful in allowing them to express their needs. The absence of moralizing or psychological misinterpretations was in sharp contrast to previous hospital experience.

This underlying basis of fellowship allowed a strength to grow in each individual and steps were taken to make changes in personality and attitude which could lead to a reduction of the pain. Advice from fellow sufferers was much more readily received than from the doctors. The respect shown and the caring help offered seemed to shine a faint light in a long dark tunnel. I am not claiming that all their pain disappeared, merely pointing out the enormous value of 'being understood' as a component in the resolution of long-term problems.

'You can never understand a man until you climb into is skin and walk around in it.'
Harper Lee, *To Kill a Mockingbird*

UNDERSTAND YOURSELF

There are many parts of this book relating to how we learn to know ourselves. The more we realize why we do these things: how we come to feel the way we do, what motivates our activities, what creates our attitudes – the more power we have to be in control of our lives and achieve our aims.

There are a variety of ways of looking at ourselves, and the following simple model is very practical and can be put to use whenever we cannot understand our limitations.

The diagram illustrates a trilogy of mechanisms we use to cope with life – thinking, feeling and behaviour. Generally, we are strong with one or two of them and weaker on the third. As an example, someone may be in touch with their feelings, good at thinking but very frightened of *doing* things. Perhaps in childhood they were ridiculed when they did something, creating a fear for future activities.

Such a person would avoid 'performing' and use logic and emotions to deal with what life offered. They are the

clients who forget to do tasks suggested in therapy, hesitant about *doing* things but very good at talking about them. Their thinking and their feelings are their *strengths* but they are also their *defences* to protect against the weaker performance part of the trio. The motto of such people is: 'Don't run in the race in case you fail.'

On the other hand, a person who is not in touch with their feelings will use logic and actions to deal with everything. Any attempt to uncover emotions will be met with logical excuses and activities. Many wives complain they never find out how their husbands feel. They prepare a cozy situation with a glass of wine by the fire to find out about the partners feelings and are met with a discussion about work or the football results.

In order to grow we need to learn more about the hidden member of the trio. This component needs support, encouragement, being vulnerable to bring it up to the level of the other two.

UNDERSTANDING – THE FACTORS INVOLVED

How can we define this 'understanding' in order to make better use of its power? Is it possible to analyze the components and propose ways to improve its capabilities?

We all know when one person is 'on our wavelength' and another is not. The feelings experienced are so different –

the first being a sense of warmth and closeness, the second an isolated feeling of being unable to express a need. In time, if misunderstandings continue, a distance develops which is difficult to bridge.

Long-term sufferers feel isolated by their problem. The receptiveness to communication is like a hedgehog rolled up into a ball. The ease of miscommunication is great and each failure adds more distance between him and 'the real world'. Understanding occurs on many levels, words alone represent the tip of the iceberg. A multitude of unconscious communications occur simultaneously, which can be unapparent to the sender and misread by the receiver. So what are the various factors necessary to understand others?

Commitment The first requirement is a commitment to try to understand. If you are in a foul mood, wrapped up in your own problems and annoyed at being disturbed, it is unlikely that you will achieve any useful understanding with someone who is seeking your help.

A patient went to his doctor late in the day with a sprained wrist. As he entered the room he had a bout of coughing. While he was coughing the doctor wrote him a prescription for a cough mixture and handed it to him. As he tried to explain that he was there for something else the doctor interrupted, and told him to take the medicine three times a day and he would be all right in a few days.

Time Time is often a factor in allowing messages to be transmitted on all levels. People will often only express their needs when they realize their listener is receptive and that takes time. In medical situations this may only occur after a number of consultations while the patient is 'sounding out' the doctor to assess whether or not the doctor can be trusted to deal with a sensitive complaint.

Mrs Wallace came to see me with a problem of anxiety. We spent an hour talking about various aspects of her difficulties. As the hour went by she gradually talked about some apparently sensitive areas. When the session was over I felt I had helped her share her problems and began to pat myself on the back for being such a good therapist. I made an appointment to see her in two weeks' time. She thanked me and walked to the door; as she left she said in a quiet voice, 'You don't think I'm going mad do you doctor?' and was gone.

Her soft comment brought me abruptly out of my self-congratulations. Here was one of the thoughts she was hoping to share with me, but was only allowed to do so as a parting gesture. She had let me know one of her deepest concerns in a way I could not reply to. I was left to wonder if this was because she was so concerned about her problem or because she felt I was not understanding enough to share it during the session. I would find the answer if she cancelled her next appointment.

The time required to gain a basis for understanding is so variable. Many people take months of cautious checking before they will unburden themselves of some of their inner concerns. A medical friend of mine told me of a patient who visited him with minimal complaints every two or three weeks over a period of two years before he was able to divulge what was worrying him.

Listening This is a major component of the art of understanding. It does not mean just hearing the spoken word – in fact it means hearing the words that are not spoken. To listen appropriately requires attention, energy, an open mind, being where the other person is coming from, tolerance and an awareness that miscommunication can occur all too easily. If someone is described as a 'good listener', it generally means they are quiet, attentive, understanding, tolerant, receptive, non-judgmental or merely wise.

We often hear what we want to hear rather than what is being said – as is the case in a busy doctor's surgery when time is always at a premium. Requests which may take time to unravel are easily missed.

'How are things at home Ted?'
'Oh, not too bad I suppose, doctor.'
'That's good Ted, now about these pills.'

The doctor doesn't want to get involved in Ted's domestic problems, even though they may be relevant to

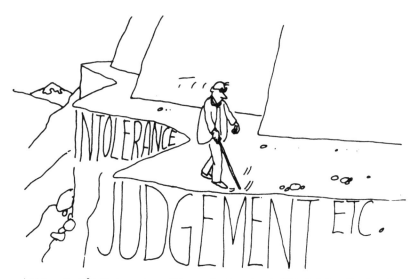

LEARNING ABOUT ATTENTIVE LISTENING IS LIKE A BLIND MAN FINDING HIS WAY DOWN A TORTUOUS PATH ...

his visit. A discussion about family matters will take much longer than prescribing tablets.

Therapeutic listening involves observing mannerisms, body language, voice intonations, slips of the tongue, choice of words, changes of expression and responses to comments. Such comments, if made with an open mind, are in themselves very helpful to someone seeking understanding. Often there is no need for advice or direction; the sharing of needs provides an avenue for increased self-worth. Being allowed to express feelings, wishes, complaints without being judged or made to feel guilty allows a release of self-imposed restriction.

Affirmation Affirmation of a person – that is confirmation of them as individuals – is a very necessary component of understanding. To affirm, declare to be true, means there is no criticism or judgment but an acceptance of the complete person – warts and all. Being reassuring and non-judgmental allows a freedom for the other person to be what he or she actually is. A confidence is created that the message given is valuable and important.

A lady recounted an interesting story to me about her childhood. She studied ballet and was very keen to do well. At the age of 15 she studied for an exam with a good teacher but one who didn't understand or affirm her. She failed the exam. Six months later after studying with another teacher, who had great belief in her ability and praised and encouraged her to do her best, she came first in the class for the whole of England. She explained that the second teacher was instrumental in helping her gain belief in herself that she *was* good and could do well in the exam.

Trust Trust is also inherent in understanding, both on the part of giver and receiver. To allow ourselves to be close enough to divulge worthwhile feelings we need to trust the listener; to be a therapeutic listener we need to trust the speaker to be voicing a real need.

Understanding, then, is the thread that helps us out of the maze. It gets stronger and easier to proceed as positive resources are affirmed and shared by the listener. The fact that a predicament is appreciated and hope suggested provides previously unrecognized energy.

TURNING POINTS

1   It is most important that people with chronic problems are understood – both by themselves and at least some other person.

2   The more you learn to understand yourself – and the problem as a part of yourself – the better able you will be to deal with it.

3   To understand someone is a skill and requires patience, non-critical listening, support and affirmation.

4   It may well be that the 'understanding component' of a therapeutic relationship is the most valuable of all the interactions that occur.

5   Learn about the weak component of your trio – thoughts, feelings and behaviour. Encourage and support that mechanism, Allow yourself to be vulnerable. Take small risks by reducing the stronger components.

6   Find someone whom you trust and can share your problem with. As you gain confidence in their ability to understand allow more and more of your inner feelings and thoughts to be expressed.

7   Sharing a problem with someone who understands diminishes the problem.

12

Fixation on the physical

'We do not see things as they are,
We see them as we are.'
Anäis Nin

'Sometimes everything is a nail to those who possess a
hammer.'

Most of us, doctors and patients alike, assume that illness
and disease have physical origins. In spite of experience
and intuition the body is blamed, investigated and treated
as the cause of the troublesome symptoms. Many times it
is the scapegoat, the messenger from the mind which
suffers a terrible fate, like the bearer of bad news in Roman
times.

To confuse matters further, the body often acts as a
decoy to divert attention from the real source of the
problem – the mind. As a result, the long-term problem will
never be resolved if all the energy is spent dealing with the
physical side of things and none spent on any psychological
aspects of the problem.

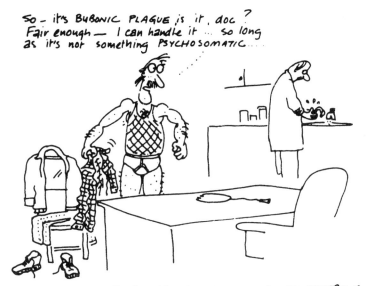

So – it's BUBONIC PLAGUE is it, doc? Fair enough — I can handle it … so long as it's not something PSYCHOSOMATIC…

WHY IS IT THAT PEOPLE ARE SO FRIGHTENED OF ACCEPTING THE POSSIBILITY THAT THEIR MIND IS PLAYING A ROLE IN THEIR PROBLEM?

One of the biggest blocks to overcoming problems is not the lack of knowledge but where this knowledge is directed. If the doctor and patient agree to avoid anything that is psychological they are agreeing to maintain the problem.

Moria has eczema and has had it for 20 years. She takes tablets and has three different creams to rub on. She scratches at night and takes tablets to help her sleep. Her eczema waxes and wanes but never goes away, and she knows it is worse when she is tense and 'uptight'. Her doctor told her six months ago she should learn to relax but she kept putting off the decision to make an appointment to learn about relaxation. When she finally plucked up courage to admit that her mind was playing a role in her problem, she rang me for an appointment. We discussed her anxieties and tensions, the role of stress in relation to her eczema and the possibility that relaxation might help.

She kept mentioning other physical treatments she had not yet tried – such as laser therapy, hot springs, mud packs, ultraviolet light and so on. At the end of the session she thought it was possible her mind could be playing a part in her problem but felt it was better to continue with the tablets as they were 'sure to help sooner or later'.

Moira represents the vast majority of people with a long-term problem. It is too great a leap to change from the physical direction to the responsibility of acquiring a new approach. This avenue is bolstered by the general attitude of the community which will support repeated tests and tablets in the hope that the 'real cure' will soon be found.

Why is it that people are so frightened of accepting the possibility that their mind is playing a role in their problem? It is as if they cling to the physical cause as a life-raft – proving it is 'not their fault'. If a leg or arm are injured it is not the person's fault, it is the fault of the leg or arm and that is acceptable. Perhaps there is a deep-seated, unconscious feeling that the mind *is* the person, and feelings of blame, guilt and responsibility for the problem are too great to bear. Have you noticed how, if someone mentions they are seeing a psychiatrist people tend to shy away, but if someone has a broken leg the chances are that they will have repeated the account of how they broke it many times?

There is a medical condition called 'referred pain' where pain is felt at a distance from the site of the problem. If the sciatic nerve is irritated at the base of the spine causing sciatica, pain may be felt in the toes. A patient complaining about painful toes is told treatment is necessary in the back some distance from the pain. We accept this as being true and the back is treated even though it is the *toes* that are feeling the pain. Why then do we seem unable to accept that something else distant from the problem, i.e. the mind, may be involved and requires attention, understanding and help?

The most common reaction, when a psychological cause is suggested, is one of disbelief, annoyance, anger and refusal to accept the possibility. It is as if labelling it as 'in the mind' means malingering, putting it on, not real, guilt-making, frightening; and so the alternative, seeking a physical cause is preferable, even if unsuccessful. We seem to be frightened of accepting a mental aspect to our problems even if the mind does need attention. Yet by remaining fixated with the physical, it is possible that we may be fixing the problem in concrete.

TURNING POINTS

1   Although your problems may be expressed as a physical one, recognize that psychological factors may be playing a major role in its maintenance.

2   Apart from the physical manifestations of your problem note the effects it is having on your confidence, attitudes and optimism.

3   Many chronic physical ailments have a basis in the mind. Until this fact is recognized improvement is unlikely. Ask yourself what part of your 'mental makeup', past, present or future, may be involved in your physical symptoms.

4   Be aware that doctors, chemists, newspapers and society will direct you to treat only the physical symptoms of your condition.

5   It is not an admission of failure or shameful to accept that your mind is playing a role in your physical problem.

13

How the other half lives – the unconscious

'My own behaviour baffles me. For I find myself not doing what I really want to do but doing what I really loathe.'
St Paul to the Romans, VII.14

As the sufferer is not intentionally maintaining the problem, we must assume there are 'hidden powers at work' which keep the merry-go-round moving in circles. We may call these powers the unconscious, although some psychiatrists believe that the unconscious is itself divided into preconscious and subconscious.

The unconscious can have an enormous effect on our daily lives. We can regard it as a *helpful* part of our mind, using many and varied methods to achieve its aims. But, often these methods do *not* achieve what is intended; they can instead create symptoms and problems. The logic and language used by our conscious mind is vastly different from that used by our unconscious ('the back of our mind') so miscommunication is inevitable. The more we learn

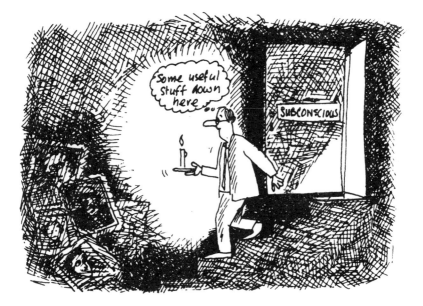

about and understand 'the other half' the better communication can be achieved, with resultant harmony and energy channelled in one direction rather than wasted in a tug-of-war.

As a simple example of the computer-like ability of the unconscious, I had arranged to play tennis on a weekend and my partner rang on Tuesday to ask the time of the game. I replied 'At one-thirty or four o'clock', and as I tried to remember, all I received from the back of my mind was 'one-thirty or four o'clock'. I couldn't make sense of my unconscious message until I checked my diary to find I was playing tennis at one-thirty on Saturday and four o'clock on Sunday. My computerized unconscious was giving me correct information, but I had not been selective enough with the question button. Just as a computer is only as good as the information fed into it, so we can improve the ability of our mind by learning more about the 'software' created for it.

NIGHTMARISH MESSAGES

The following case history of a man suffering from nightmares illustrates how the unconscious attempts to help us, often unsuccessfully. As nightmares occur while a person is asleep the mind is obviously beyond conscious control. Equally, they can be analyzed without the temptation of looking for physical causes.

Scott is a 23-year-old salesman and had had nightmares or 'night terrors' for many years. He was only vaguely aware of them but his mother, a light sleeper, was alert all night for the screams and disturbances which emanated from Scott's bedroom. His nightmares took the form of shouting, getting out of bed, crouching in the corner and knocking over furniture in terror. The content of the dreams often involved someone chasing him to hurt him, or an animal running after him.

He had sought help from a lay hypnotherapist, an acupuncturist and counselling. There were some temporary improvements but the nightmares returned and caused disturbances most nights of the week.

Scott's father was in the RAF and was transferred constantly, so as a child Scott had changed schools many times. He was small for his age and constantly bullied as the new boy in the class, going through long periods of fear and misery. His younger brother was taller and more successful at most things and Scott lived in his shadow.

After leaving school, Scott joined the RAF to please his father but decided it was not the career for him and left after a year to take up a job as salesman which he now held.

This move was very traumatic as it involved going against his father's wishes.

He was a quiet, gentle boy with a shy, appealing nature and an honest open personality, troubled by his problem and its effect on his parents who were naturally very concerned. He was worried that he might hurt himself since on one occasion, while trying to escape his nocturnal pursuer, he had crashed into a window and broken it.

In order to understand what message his unconscious mind was trying to send, via the dreams, I taught him a form of deep relaxation so that he could 'talk to his inner mind' and learn more about its nocturnal activities. He sat with his eyes closed, relaxed his breathing and allowed himself to imagine he was going into the back of his mind. During the first session he learnt to 'turn off' a little and over the next few sessions he practised 'getting in touch' with himself by allowing any thoughts or feelings to drift into his mind without trying to analyze or understand them.

On the fifth visit he said he could see a large hole in front of him and he was trying to get out of it. I suggested he helped that Scott, in the back of his mind, out of the hole. When he did this we talked about filling in the hole so there would be no more problems. As he started to fill in the hole he exclaimed, 'there are more of me down there'. I asked him to allow them out and he sat for many minutes without moving, his eyes closed, apparently intent on what he was visualizing in his mind.

'There are hundreds of them coming out' he murmured, 'in soldiers' uniforms or RAF uniforms, all shapes and sizes, many of them are very small.'

We discussed what was happening and it appeared that the 'little people' were Scott during his various stages of growing up. They had all suffered fear and were hiding in the hole. Some were in Roman togas, others in the red uniforms of Wellington's troops. He allowed them to gather around him on the ground surrounding the hole, and after half-an-hour had thousands of little Scotts quietly standing around him.

As an hour had passed, I asked him to open his eyes to interpret what all this meant to him. He said he really didn't know but felt a lot better; he thought they may have represented the times when he had been bullied or frightened. When I asked about his father's attitude towards him he replied, 'He's always putting me down' (the hole). I told him to spend half an hour a day 'freeing the Scotts' from the hole and allowing them to join him. During the next week he only had one night when a disturbance occurred and that was minimal.

At his last session we discussed his experiences during the week. He said he was feeling more relaxed and free and had 'liberated' thousands from the hole but they kept coming. He tried filling in the hole containing his 'unwanted fear' but they climbed up a fire escape on the side. I asked him to go back to the relaxed state and talk to the soldiers to find out if they were responsible for his nightmares and why. He replied that they were giving him the bad dreams because they were 'mad at him for not letting them out during the day'. When we discussed this, it seemed he had always ignored his feelings – not accepted them, but kept them in check – 'down the hole'.

When trying to find out the aim of the nightmares it appeared they had punishment function. Even though their method was not working (in that he was often unaware of his dreams), the punishment was filtering through to his parents by causing them concern. As well as the small soldiers there was a single Scott with his hands raised as if asking to be let out. When he was helped out he became a baby whom Scott cuddled. On questioning the baby it appeared that his presence represented a difficult birth, and 'he couldn't breathe down there'. As an hour had again passed with Scott sitting motionless with his eyes closed, I asked him to come out of the relaxed state to discuss his thoughts. He commented that indeed his mother had experienced a very difficult delivery with him and he had required oxygen and that as a result of his condition he was not handled or fed for 24 hours.

Just before he left, Scott gave me a poem he had written some time previously. It seems to be giving some subtle messages relating to the workings in the back of his mind.

> And of this place
> And of a dream
> And deep inside
> A man called queen
> He kept a secret
> For days and nights
> And felt the danger
> And the fright
> It was a kiss
> That could have seen
> It was a mouth
> That could have been
> A secret kept
> Beneath a grave
> A curse of which
> He was a slave.

A summary of Scott's case may give some insight into the workings of his unconscious mind:

- he had an insecure childhood, moving school, small of

stature, constantly bullied;
- he felt constantly 'put down' by his father, inferior to his younger brother and unable to express his feelings;
- he had nightmares for some years and was only partially aware of them, but they were disturbing to the other members of his family;
- his birth was traumatic;
- he learnt, via relaxation and 'communication with the back of his mind', about 'little Scotts forced to remain down a hole' who claimed to be responsible for his nightmares;
- the 'stated aim' of the nightmares was to punish him (and his family) for being unaware of his feelings;
- the birth experience may have been depicted as the 'babe suffocating in the hole';
- by communicating with the back of his mind and accepting his feelings the nightmares diminished;
- by spending time during the day 'talking to himself' nocturnal messages were no longer necessary;
- the need for self-punishment diminished as he became aware of his dreams' intentions.

These statements are all hypothetical. The only facts we have are that Scott had nightmares for many years which abruptly ceased when he interpreted images which occurred to him when he was in a relaxed state.

I believe this illustrates some aspects of the workings of the unconscious mind and how interpreting the messages may minimize unpleasant symptoms. The logic of the unconscious (prehistoric soldiers, babies talking) is vastly different from conscious logic.

From the cases of Scott and other patients, I believe it is possible to state that:

- many physical and psychological symptoms can be viewed as messages from the unconscious;
- some form of unconscious communication to decipher the symptoms may relieve them;
- the unconscious can be thought of as a beneficial part of the mind although the results may be the reverse;
- the length of time required to 'decode' messages varies enormously;
- supportive help in translating the messages is necessary;
- an 'open mind' to any interpretation is essential;
- a 'ripple effect' often occurs in other areas of life leading to a more relaxed and confident personality;

Assuming the unconscious mind is playing a major role in long-term problems, whether they are in relationships or in physical or psychological illness, it is important to achieve an understanding of that role if the problem is to be resolved. By ignoring this factor the problem is often augmented in order for the unconscious to have its 'message heard', for example indigestion relating to overwork and stress may lead to a peptic ulcer if the message to alter the lifestyle is ignored.

By widening the parameters of our mind we increase the energy available to resolve problems. The more our unconscious is understood the more we can harness the vast potential stored there.

TURNING POINTS

1   Be aware that the unconscious exists and that it exerts a great influence on your life.

2   The presence of the unconscious is made known in dreams, slips of the tongue, body language and actions that you make that are apparently beyond your control.

3   Getting in touch with your unconscious will provide you with a greater understanding of your behaviour and emotions.

4   Learning from your symptoms and unconscious messages is preferable to blaming yourself for failures and mistakes.

5   Read some of the many books available to improve your knowledge of the unconscious.

14

Different levels controlling behaviour

'If the errand boy is incompetent the whole business may collapse.'

One way to analyse our behaviour is to view it as a result of influences coming from different levels of our mind.

For example, Mary is 45 and 5 stone overweight. She is overweight because:

Top Level   She eats too much and doesn't do enough exercise.

Next Level   She is lonely and needs comfort for her loneliness.

Next Level   She lacks confidence and uses eating to avoid challenges.

Next Level   She uses her excess weight as an excuse for her failures in life.

Next Level   As a child she was constantly criticized by her parents and resorted to food to cope with the pain.

There are many reasons why Mary is overweight. *All these reasons are true*, and they are acting on her at different levels. Each level contains experiences and emotions resulting in the weight problem.

Statistically it has been shown that diets, eating less, does not have long-term results with many overweight people. This is because the problem is only tackled on one level – the top 'eat less' level – leaving all the other levels to continue to influence us.

For any long-term problem – one that is not resolved by dealing with it on the most superficial level – we need to examine the conflicts occurring elsewhere in the mind. This is often called the 'hidden agenda' and applies when we hear the comment 'the more things change the more they stay the same'.

Lucy and Tom have been married for 2 years and are always fighting. Their relationship at home and with friends always ends in tears and anger.

On examining the patterns involved we find:

Level 1   Lucy is angry with Tom because he is often home late from work.

Level 2   Lucy is an insecure person and waiting for Tom heightens this feeling of low self-esteem.

Level 3   Lucy worries Tom may be having an affair.

Level 4   Five years ago Tom had an affair and this has not been properly resolved.

Level 5   Lucy's first marriage ended because her husband left her for another woman. Lucy is still bitter and hurt from this experience.

Level 6   Lucy's parents divorced when she was 10.

Her father left her mother for another woman.

Level 7   Lucy has a deep and frightening need to be loved. She is angry at herself for having this need and angry with Tom for neglecting this need and coming home late.

By observing this situation it becomes understandable why it is not being resolved. The different levels are not being addressed and the resulting arguments and tears are the tip of the iceberg.

Therapy, counselling, supportive listening involves dealing with conflicts at deeper levels. This process is called 'working through unresolved conflicts'. As each conflict is discussed it can be released leaving the lower levels free from problems that may influence present behaviour.

Often the deeper messages are 'I need to be loved' or 'I'm no good'. These messages will undermine any efforts directed at more superficial levels and need to be addressed to allow progress.

TURNING POINTS

1   Write down an unresolved situation which has been present for some time.
2   Make a list of different levels that may be involved in preventing resolution.
3   Focus your attention on one level that you can do something about, and do it.
4   Over a period of time notice the benefit created by diminishing the conflict on that level.

15

It's about time

'The now, the here, through which all future
plunges into the past.'
James Joyce, *Ulysses*

'Time isn't always a question of length;
it's a question of depth.'

'Time present and time past
Are both perhaps present in time future,
And time future contained in time past.'
T.S. Eliot, *Burnt Norton*

Every cook knows there are ingredients, however small, that are essential to the flavour of the finished dish. If these ingredients are misjudged or forgotten a culinary delight becomes a disaster. It may be a pinch of salt or a clove of garlic, but all the effort of sweating over a hot stove will not achieve the desired result without them. Time (not thyme) is such an ingredient in dealing with difficulties and its role is vital.

LIFE IS NOW

Life exists in the present and in the present alone. We may bring the past or future into existence by thoughts, attitudes or expressions, but we *live* in the present. To a greater or lesser extent we flavour (or sour) our immediate experiences with memories or wishful thinking, and the proportion of the future or past ingredient determines the energy available for the present.

Although we are physically rooted in the present, our minds may take us on a time journey in either direction. Our psychic make-up determines whether we are mentally looking over our shoulder or craning our necks towards the future. Gurdjieff wrote: 'How shattering during a war to view a truck loaded up with crutches on its way to a military hospital – crutches for limbs that had not been blown off yet.'

There are people who are always anticipating the destination and ignoring the journey. The present is swallowed up as a passing phase and the mind is absorbed by what is

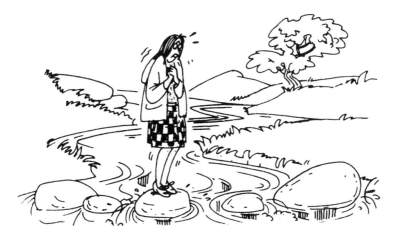

in store. These *anticipators* live in a fantasy world of expectations, hopes and dreams. Some anticipators are *future worriers* and act as if stranded on a stepping stone in a stream believing they will fall in if they move. Any suggestion concerning the future is met with repeated phrases beginning with 'What if . . .?' Their ability to create disasters out of nothing rivals the creativity of great artists, but always with a negative outcome. As they are constantly worried about things that are yet to happen the energy left for the present is reduced.

Due to their future worry these people are often able to create the disasters they anticipate, which reinforces more future predictions of gloom and doom. Their merry-go-round is occurring in the future and dragging them into it as a whirlpool sucks everything in its vicinity down to the bottom. Any forward progress is blocked by the wall of future fear and unless this barrier is lowered, logic and supportive explanations fall on deaf ears.

'I feel really lousy because I'm sure it's going to rain next week and my party will be a complete flop.'

'Although a rise is long overdue I can't ask the boss because he is sure to refuse and may sack me for being impertinent.'

'You ask me to go swimming to lose weight. What if everyone in the pool laughs at me?'

This 'what if' syndrome is a very powerful force perpetuating the circular pattern of remaining stationary.

Anticipators often miss out on the present by their future fantasy life. While having soup, thoughts of the main course flavour their palate; the steak is swallowed in a haze of crème caramel; the aroma of after-dinner coffee taints their dessert. They are never 'where it's at' but always 'where it will be'. They have an incessant urge to move on, little realizing that they are going nowhere, except to where they are not – the future.

Difficulties also arise when the present is relegated to a secondary position by the hopeful belief 'won't it be wonderful when . . .', without steps being taken to ensure this happens. This constant inability to do something about the present, because of the magical future when it will be wonderful, enables time to march by unchallenged and the future to remain as a carrot firmly attached to the stick tantalizing the donkey, but forever out of reach. As it is said in the Bible, it is enough to live each day as it comes:

'Take therefore no thought for the morrow; for the morrow shall take thought for the things of itself. Sufficient unto the day is the evil thereof.'

St Matthew VI, 34

LIVING IN THE PAST

'Even God cannot change the past.'

Aristotle

The anticipators are not the only people to ignore or belittle the present. Some people are forever looking over their shoulders at things gone by. These people, the *reminiscers*, also live a fantasy life out of reality. For them the photo albums, recollections, yarns about 'the good old days', help the present to become a future fairyland to be 'put up with' as a distracting inconvenience, limiting the time spent in the heyday of 'real' life.

This past prescription may be a pleasant dream providing a balm for present wounds or an excuse for failure, but the past is past – unchangeable. If you waste energy

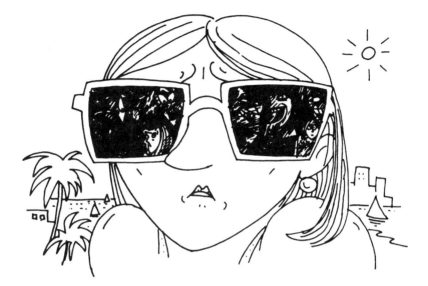

blaming past events for present-day problems, progress in all areas of your life will be minimal.

We cannot change the past but we can alter the effect the past has on us (see chapter 21). Previous experiences, painful and frightening, colour our present-day views as sunglasses filter out the sun. Although we cannot alter the actual happenings we can learn to appreciate the bias they have on our attitudes and confidence and spend time allowing the past to drift back to where it belongs – in the past.

Asking yourself the following question may help you to see if past influences are limiting your actions: 'Am I acting in an up-to-date way to deal with present-day situations or am I being limited by childish behaviour similar to past performances?'

One patient severely reprimanded in childhood had present-day reactions of the type, 'I can't stand being shouted at. I've left many jobs because people raised their voices at me. I think it is not right for them to do that and I just won't be talked to in that way'. The past was so discolouring his present that limitations occurred in many areas of his life. He needed to learn that the situation was vastly different to the childhood he had so vividly and painfully stored in his mind. He also needed to realize that his potential for response was much greater than when he was a child.

DIFFERENT PEOPLE, DIFFERENT TIMING

'It will take time – your own time.'
Dr Milton Erickson, American psychiatrist

Time measured by the clock is standardized throughout the world. A minute in London is identical to a minute in Tokyo, but internal time measured by the mind varies greatly from person to person; we all require our own timing to do things, change, face difficulties. Some people approach problems as they arise, others need to build up their confidence to 'feel right' before proceeding.

Being told to attempt something before you are ready may well result in failure whereas success would have been the outcome if the timing was appropriate. As an old yoga teacher once said. 'Think of yourself as an explorer going into new territory. A wise explorer goes slowly for he never knows what may be around the bend.'

Understanding your own and your partner's and colleagues' internal clocks and accepting them may prevent a great deal of conflict. Allowing for this difference provides a basis for acknowledgment of individuality. Comments such as 'Come on, I could have done that in half the time' do not necessarily achieve the desired result. Allowing people to do things 'their own way' incorporates time in the formula used.

It is as if we all have metronomes inside our minds dictating the rate at which we think, act and respond to situations. As they are ticking away at different rates the responses for individuals will vary. Recognizing our own speed and accepting it will allow a greater peace of mind than trying to keep pace with someone else whose 'metronome' is set at a different rate. The picture of the nervous husband chain smoking, pacing the floor, looking at his watch waiting for his wife to finish dressing for their dinner party, depicts the tension generated by different timing mechanisms.

Many words, thoughts, experiences sink into the unconscious and need time to 'grow and mature' to provide energy and resources to cope with future difficulties. Some children are slow learners, but become mathematical wizards in later life; some babies don't walk until they are two, but are competing in marathons in their teens. Accepting and making allowances for such differences in timing, both in ourselves and others, gives individual potential the best circumstances in which to develop.

MAKE TIME FOR YOURSELF

'No hordes of people pestering me
Trampling over my time.'
Rabindranath Tagore, *In the Eyes of the Peacock*

We spend most of our lives learning, using, understanding and giving our time to objects, people and activities outside ourselves; yet how much time do we actually spend thinking about or understanding the most important person of all – ourselves?

It seems as if there is an unspoken but powerful commandment in the Western world 'Thou must not delve into the mind, think too seriously or analyze thyself' which prevents us exploring the dusty corridors and pathways multiplying in the back of the mind as we grow. Anyone who meditates, does yoga, practises Zen Buddhism or self-hypnosis or proposes discussions about behaviour or the psyche is regarded as a bit strange – someone to be wary of.

It is acceptable to take pills, alcohol, drugs, have an operation, work too hard, ignore or just accept ill feelings rather than learn more about the workings of the mind by spending time thinking about yourself. A strange word 'selfish' seems to creep in as the argument against any time spent relaxing. Time spent on others – children, spouse, in-laws, charities, church, the cat, canary or gerbil – assumes priority and two minutes' relaxation in the bath before bed is felt as over-indulgent and not to be allowed.

This is all nonsense! Spending time on yourself is one of the most basic and essential requirements for achieving the potential you possess. This potential can be guided in any direction you wish – towards your family, making money, being successful at sport or even raising pedigree gerbils, but unless time is spent on yourself, your potential will not be realized.

So many people find the time not to find the time to learn about themselves or provide tranquillity in their daily hectic life. The amount of time required may be as little as 15 or 20 minutes a day spent relaxing – 'being not doing', valuable as insurance against illness and restoring the imbalance imposed by 'progress'. It is not a lot to ask on behalf of the body but to many it appears an insurmountable task.

Think of time as currency, and the biblical 'three score

years and ten' as your bank balance. By taking a little time and trouble, you may be able to invest it and live longer and more healthily. Without care, however, as you get older you may find your currency devalued, leaving you with no suitable pension fund of health.

TURNING POINTS

1 Take time into account when anticipating any change.
2 Check on your own timing and that of your partner and others to whom you relate.
3 You live in the *present*; assess how much of you is involved in the past or future.
4 Increase the proportion of your time spent in the 'here and now'.
5 Allow time for yourself. This will provide abilities to spend time on other things.

16

The diversionary tactics
of stress

'Anxiety is the watch dog of the mind warning us all is not
well. But if our guardian runs wild our troubles grow a
hundred-fold.'
Ainslie Meares, MD, *A Way of Doctoring*

'Approximately 80 per cent of the people who walk into
doctors' offices are there because of stress-related
diseases.'
Californian Institute of Technology, 1980

A sniper firing into a crowd creates pandemonium and
havoc. People terrified of being hit by the bullets run in all
directions, seeking cover and security from the hidden
marksman. After reaching safety, time and effort are spent
uncovering the source of the bullets to prevent further
injury.

Stress is such a sniper and inflicts damage to areas of the

body distant from the source of the problem. We generally focus attention on where the 'bullet strikes' and so allow the sharpshooter to go scot-free. No organ or anatomical site is safe; the targets may change or the damage to the original area may just be increased.

If I were to defend the sniper stress, I could say it is attempting to bring to conscious awareness problems that exist in the 'mind-body' system. These problems may be related to external conditions in the present or to those stored in the back of the mind from the past. Painful ammunition is essential because previous messages have gone unheeded.

Conditions related to stress cover the whole spectrum of medical complaints. As a medical student I learnt that syphilis was the universal imitator; almost any condition from blindness to ruptured arteries could be caused by syphilis. Stress has now taken that role and is behind many of the physical problems afflicting patients today.

Hospital skin clinics are full of patients suffering from chronic skin complaints – painful, itchy, unsightly, weeping and disruptive to their lives. These conditions grumble on for years crying out for help yet the sniper stress, using the skin as the target, goes unnoticed. Creams, tablets, lotions, heat lamps, are all used as remedies for the target organ without attention being paid to where the bullets are coming from.

If underlying stress is not discovered it often increases its intensity, as the following case-history illustrates.

Jonathon is an overworked salesman, underpaid and angry at his work situation. He is a born worrier and inwardly digests his frustration and annoyance at the many confrontations he faces with his boss at work. His wife complains he 'never leaves the office', bringing the problems home with him and continually worrying about all the frustrations besetting him. Whenever she asks him to relax and not worry an argument ensues, he accuses her of spending too much, so causing him to have to work harder, and she bursts into tears.

The sniper stress sits on the sidelines confident he will be called in to help Jonathon by providing painful messages; he chooses Jonathon's stomach as his target. Jonathon develops indigestion and complains about the constant gnawing pain in his abdomen. He receives sympathy from his wife and antacid tablets from his doctor.

The pain continues so he goes on a bland diet of milk and sops. The sniper sighs and continues to attack until a barium meal is ordered which shows no ulcer; a gastro-scopy (looking into the stomach by a small telescope through the mouth) is performed, indicating a red, angry, irritated stomach lining with increased acidity.

Jonathon is advised to take things easier, have a holiday, a rest. He curses to himself that people do not understand that he can't take a holiday because of all his commitments.

The sniper decides it is time to increase the message, the pain gets worse and as months go by Jonathon begins to look haggard and unwell, loses weight and becomes irritable. Another barium meal is performed, this time showing a duodenal ulcer. Stronger tablets are prescribed with the threat of an operation if the ulcer doesn't heal.

During all this time, although Jonathon, his wife and the doctor are aware of the sniper in the background as the underlying cause, no-one listens to the message or advises Jonathon in such a way that our anti-hero can go off duty.

RECOGNIZING STRESS

One of the biggest hurdles confronting us in chronic conditions is to recognize the role stress is playing and focus our attention on it. The stress factor may be related to existing conditions at home, work, relationships, finances, and so on, or it may be a persistent message from the past caused by fear, guilt or anger that has not been resolved.

Understanding the source of the stress and developing techniques to deal with it by relaxation, hypnosis or a build-up of assertive skills may be the correct attitude to many symptoms represented as physical illnesses. Unfortunately, it is a typical 'Catch-22' situation, where those who need help to deal with tension, anxiety and worry are the least likely to accept it.

By understanding your body better – recognizing your feelings, attitudes and restrictions, your peculiarities, strengths and weaknesses – you can learn about the symptoms and the part they are playing in your life. By finding the areas of stress and tension, whether they are stored in the back of your mind or confront you daily, you will be able to determine the direction of the sniper's bullets.

MIND READING

Many people cause stress for themselves by a practice I call 'mind reading'. They are constantly concerned what other people will think about them.

'Oh, I couldn't go to the pictures. If I got a panic and wanted to get out, all the people in the theatre will think I'm terrible.'

'When I meet people for the first time I just go to jelly because I know they think I'm hopeless.'

This constant reference to what people think causes limitations and tension. The sad but true fact of the matter is that *people don't care*, they are too busy with their own problems to be overly concerned by the minutiae of our lives. Secondly, how will we ever know what other people think? If we ask them they are unlikely to tell us if it is critical.

I strongly advise my patients not to get into the mind reading game. It can never be verified and usually is restricting rather than supportive.

DEALING WITH STRESS

Facing up to stressful factors is generally the most important step towards dealing with them. It is natural for us to avoid, ignore and run away from painful and unpleasant things; as a result they tend to grow and become worse.

A 30-year-old man came to see me, complaining that he was constantly frightened by a dragon-like creature in the back of his mind. This fear had been present for two years and caused him lack of sleep, irritability, family rows and headaches.

I asked him how he knew about the dragon and he explained it was always there in the back of his mind, causing him to feel frightened all over his body.

'What does it look like?' I asked.

'I don't know, I'm too frightened to look. It is as if it is in a room and I've kept the door tightly closed.'

'Let's have a look at him, while you are safe with me in the surgery.'

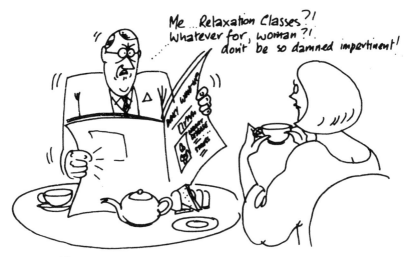

THOSE WHO NEED HELP TO DEAL WITH TENSION, ANXIETY AND WORRY ARE THE LEAST LIKELY TO ACCEPT IT...

'No way! I couldn't do that – it's too terrifying.'

'OK. When I see you next week we will take a peek by gradually opening the door knowing we can always close it.'

He reluctantly agreed and spent the week in fear and trepidation, wondering what he would encounter. At the next meeting he was very anxious, his knuckles shining white as he gripped the arms of the chair.

'Close your eyes and imagine that room with the dragon in it. When you can see it with the door closed nod your head.'

After a few minutes he cautiously nodded his head.

'OK. Now open the door a fraction and peer through. What can you see?'

'It's dark. I can't see anything.'

'Good. Open it a few more inches and allow some light

in. Can you see anything yet?'

'No. The room seems empty.'

'Good. Shine a little more light in until you can see the whole room.'

'Yes. I can see him in the corner.'

'What does he look like?'

'Oh! He's a frightened little boy crouching in the corner very afraid. He looks like me when I was very young!'

Recently I needed the help of a dental hygienist to deal with sensitive teeth and receding gums. I was becoming long in the tooth! For the previous 40 years I had brushed my teeth and attended a dentist regularly and had thought that that was quite enough to ensure dental health. As she looked in my mouth the hygienist started using battleground terminology, referring to the dreaded enemy 'plaque'. Terms like 'fighting', 'destruction', 'erosion' and 'invasion' were floated across my gaping mouth. I had neglected to do adequate battle with this invasive foe and it had been winning the war against my poor gums for all those years.

Desperate treatment was required to put the invader to flight and so commenced hour-long sessions of self-defence – scraping, brushing, flossing, cleaning to regain control. I was told to spend half-an-hour each day brushing correctly and flossing as plaque is always present and will build up as soon as one's back is turned.

It seems to me that there is a similar comparison to stress and its effects although they are neither so obvious nor so discernible. If we ignore the build-up of stress and its bodily symptoms, it will be the victor and we, our minds and bodies, will be the vanquished.

Just as regular attention to dental hygiene is essential to prevent gum disease, so relaxation, awareness of stressful messages and the building of self-confidence are important to protect our body and all the intricate devices that keep us healthy.

Hypnosis is a useful tool to uncover stress snipers dwelling in the back of the mind. Using hypnotic techniques it is possible to view past problems from a safe distance, allowing daylight and the fresh air of the present to dissolve them. Often we are too close to a situation to see it clearly. If you stand too near a painting, all you see is a mess of colour and brush-strokes, but if you move away from it the whole picture can be enjoyed and understood. Try to remember this in dealing with your own problems. Counselling can be useful in this way, because an outsider sees problems in a different perspective – we are too close to the 'picture' of our lives.

Building confidence and self-esteem provides us with an arsenal to deal with the sniper. If the condition is irritating, painful or depressing it will drain our confidence, reducing our resources by constant worry.

Relaxation exercises and techniques play a worthwhile role in lessening muscle tension and mental anxiety, providing space and freedom from worry for a period of time – an oasis on the desert journey. Learning to breathe slowly and quietly, relax muscles, visualize and have time for yourself, all provide energy to cope with commitments. Fitting these techniques into the daily schedule gives a balance to the hectic pace of modern society; just as brushing your teeth daily prevents decay, so the relaxation exercises can reduce stress.

If you can make use of your problem or discomfort to learn more about yourself, you will reduce the power of the problem, so enabling you to grow and expand in other, positive directions.

TURNING POINTS

1 Stress plays a major role in causing or maintaining long-term problems.
2 The effects of stress can be many and varied.
3 Learning to recognize any long-term problem as being stress-related is the first step.
4 Check how often you play the 'mind reading game'. Focus on steps to reduce it when with other people.
5 Identifying the symptoms as messages gives you some power over the problem.
6 Learn to minimise the effects of the stress by relaxation techniques, hypnosis or reading suitable books (see reading list).
7 Make a commitment to spend 20 minutes a day doing battle with the sniper stress.

17

A breath of fresh air – hyperventilation

Air pollution is a problem, but it may well be the *way* we breathe and not *what* we breathe that underlies our illness. Of all the self-inflicted causes of long-term problems who would suspect the most basic of human functions – breathing – to be the culprit of a multitude of chronic illnesses?

It is becoming more and more apparent that *hyperventilation* is a factor in many symptoms which find their way to the doctor's surgery. Insidious in onset and unnoticed by doctor and patient alike, it underlies many problems and undermines their resolution. Hyperventilation means breathing more air in and out than is necessary. It is an incorrect breathing habit often learnt early in life. It is impossible to state what percentage of the population suffer from this habit but the more it is investigated the more common it seems to be.

We breathe in two ways:

- With our diaphragm – the horizontal sheet of muscle between our chest and abdomen – which is raised and lowered to control the inspiration and expiration of air. This is the basic mechanism used for air exchange when we are at rest.
- Using our chest muscles – the muscles between the ribs – to raise and lower the chest wall sucking in and blowing out air. This method is used when we need extra oxygen for exercise or effort.

Breathing is the basic system of the human body. As we breathe in (inspiration), the lungs extract oxygen from the air and pass it on to the bloodstream which carries it to all parts of the body. The oxygen is necessary for the survival of cells and tissues in the body which are soon damaged if the oxygen level falls. Breathing out (expiration) rids the body of excess air and the waste product carbon dioxide, produced by the different functions of the tissues and cells.

The carbon dioxide in the body can affect the different tissues in different ways and the body has delicate mechanisms to maintain the level of carbon dioxide in the blood within normal limits. But this is where the problem starts! If the amount of carbon dioxide falls below a certain level many symptoms may occur. If we breathe with our chest when we are at rest we get rid of more carbon dioxide than is necessary, the blood level falls and unfortunate symptoms are produced.

Some of the symptoms associated with hyperventilation are:

- *heart* – palpitations, tachycardia (fast heart-beat), chest pains, irregular heart beats;
- *nerves* – dizziness, fainting, headaches, numbness,

blurred vision, intolerance of bright lights or noise, tension, anxiety, panic attacks;
- *breathing* – coughing, asthma, sighing, yawning;
- *bowels* – flatulence, belching, abdominal pains;
- *muscles* – cramps, twitches;
- *general* – weakness, tiredness, sweating, sleep problems, exhaustion, a feeling of depersonalization (being outside oneself).

HOW DOES HYPERVENTILATION DEVELOP?

There are many avenues that lead to this condition so it may not be apparent how it develops in each individual case. It is a *learned* problem, so at some stage we have changed from natural breathing with the diaphragm to chest breathing and continued with this incorrect habit.

Being anxious or under stress makes us breathe more rapidly as a 'fight or flight' reaction developed thousands of years ago to help early humans deal with the physical dangers surrounding them. This reaction is now inappropriate, but is still set in motion in stressful situations.

The habit might have started as a result of a stressful situation in childhood which has continued into adulthood. Perhaps the stressful conditions face us now and the breathing pattern is a direct response to them. Singers, musicians, army personnel, dancers, and others in similar careers are taught to overbreathe and find it difficult to lose the habit. Some childhood illnesses, such as bronchitis or asthma, may have been the cause.

People who are chronically tense maintain their abnormal breathing pattern as if in a response to continuous fear. If symptoms develop these cause further concern and so a vicious cycle of hyperventilation symptoms causing more hyperventilation arises.

HOW DO WE KNOW IF WE ARE HYPERVENTILATING?

This may be very simple. If we breathe with our chest muscles when we are at rest, our chest will move up and down; if we are breathing with the diaphragm our abdomen will move in and out.

Sit in a chair and place one hand on your chest and one on your abdomen. Notice which one moves while you are at rest. If your chest moves you are a hyperventilator, if your abdomen moves you are not.

You may need to be observed by someone who understands this condition to find out if you are overbreathing or not, as in some cases the movement is very slight and is not obvious to the untrained observer. Sometimes blood tests to determine the level of carbon dioxide may be required to confirm the diagnosis, or the symptoms themselves may indicate hyperventilation as the culprit.

The breathing pattern of the hyperventilator is often shallow, rapid, irregular and associated with sighing. The pattern varies with emotional needs rather than the physical demands of effort. In most cases there is no obvious puffing and panting; it may be a very gentle alteration in the breathing pattern which causes problems by its continuation day and night.

Brenda is a 38-year-old mother of two. She has felt exhausted since the death of her mother three years ago. She drags herself around at work, doing the housework and preparing the meals. She has no energy or enthusiasm for herself, her family, her work or the world around her. Most days she has a sharp and unexplained chest pain.

She has seen many doctors and had many tests and tablets but her condition has persisted. On attending a hospital she was seen by the occupational therapist who noticed she was hyperventilating.

She was taught how to breathe with her abdomen, given relaxation exercises and time off work to adjust to a different outlook. She was advised to go swimming regularly and allow her children to take more responsibility for themselves.

When seen again three weeks later she claimed she had not felt so good for years, her chest pain had stopped, there were still many worries but she allowed them to go over her head and her breathing was much more relaxed and abdominal. She felt as if she was in control once more.

Lizzie, a 24-year-old student, was always hassling with her flatmate and in a constant state of agitation. For many months she had been tired and suffered from chest pains, dizzy spells, pins and needles and migraine headaches. Nothing she did seemed to alter her predicament and as time went by she became worried it would be with her forever. She was hyperventilating to a marked extent. Her chest was heaving in and out and there were constant sighs during the interview.

She was instructed how to alter her breathing to a calmer, more relaxed, abdominal style, but found it too difficult to comprehend during the first session. She became confused which only added to her anxiety. She took a holiday for two weeks and on her return was able to master the normal breathing pattern.

When seen a month later she felt much better, more relaxed and comfortable. There had only been an occasional chest pain and they were reduced by concentrating on her abdominal breathing. She was much more tolerant and able to accept her flatmate's behaviour.

HOW IS HYPERVENTILATION TREATED?

It is important to recognize that overbreathing exists and may therefore be a factor in maintaining unpleasant symptoms. Other aspects need to be investigated and treated while the breathing is being corrected. If the hyperventilation continues it may undermine any improvement in other aspects of a chronic problem.

Anxiety and tension may be corrected by relaxation exercises, counselling, meditation or yoga, support and understanding. Hypnosis may be useful in providing insight and building confidence. But re-education of 'the bad breathing' habit is necessary to restore the carbon dioxide level to a normal value. This may take time as the old pattern may be difficult to break.

It is necessary to spend time each day retraining the breathing pattern in a relaxed manner. Do this by lying down or sitting in a comfortable chair with one hand on the chest and the other on the abdomen. By concentrating on the regular movement of the abdomen while maintaining the chest in a stationary position, the breathing can be directed towards normality. But don't try to force it or try too hard as that will add to the problem. It may even be necessary to have supervision from a physiotherapist to guide and support the relearning.

Being aware of the breathing pattern is the first major step towards improving it. During the day noticing whether the abdomen or chest are moving during breathing allows the possibility of change. As we breathe many thousands of times a day it is understandable how the smallest increase in rate or volume of each breath will cause a major change in carbon dioxide level in the blood.

Although many relaxation techniques such as yoga, meditation or hypnosis focus on the breathing pattern as a basic factor for achieving tranquillity and comfort, you may find that just thinking about your breathing is all that is necessary for things to improve.

TURNING POINTS

1 Hyperventilation underlies the maintenance of many long-term problems.
2 If you have some of the symptoms described you may well be a hyperventilator.
3 Check your breathing by placing one hand on the chest and one on the abdomen as described.
4 Either on your own or with the help of a trained physiotherapist alter your breathing pattern to be slow, shallow and abdominal.
5 Allow time for 'ups and downs' to occur during the relearning process and don't be worried by them.

18

How are your feelings?

Our emotions (feelings) form a bridge between our mind and body, indeed our emotions play a major role in our enjoyment or otherwise of life, yet our understanding of them often leaves a lot to be desired. If only we would listen to them and learn from them they would provide us with a wealth of information about dealing with everyday situations.

If you are unaware of your feelings you limit your resources dramatically. This lack of awareness may be due to any one (or more) of a multitude of causes. Often it is a defence mechanism against being hurt as shown by the lines of a poem written by a depressed patient:

> 'Overwhelmed by despair
> I stopped feeling.'

FEELINGS AS AN INTERNAL BODY LANGUAGE

Most large commercial organizations have two telephone systems: one for the outside world and one for inter-departmental communications. In the same way, the body has its own internal communication system which, like any other system, can malfunction, so providing a basis for long-term problems.

The system involves three steps:

- a bodily sensation is felt – there are hundreds of examples such as pain, tightness, tingling, blushing, hollow feeling, heaviness, aches and pressure.
- these sensations are registered and 'interpreted' as emotions which we then describe to ourselves or others as feelings: I feel depressed, angry, hungry, tense, worried, frightened, happy and so on;
- we act or react to the 'interpretation' – that is we express our 'feeling' by doing something appropriate such as eating or having a temper tantrum or taking defensive action.

Sadly, as you will have realized from the case histories in this book and perhaps even from your own experience, many, many people do not understand these messages and ignore or misinterpret them. All too often we act or react according to the interpretation and not the *feeling*; as many feelings are misinterpreted we follow the wrong path which may be a circular one. Learning to decode our feelings correctly will allow us to make use of our bodily sensations to grow and expand our world.

Some time ago I visited a friend's farm which had a septic tank. There was a terrible smell of sewage in the area where the septic tank was buried. When I asked my friend what

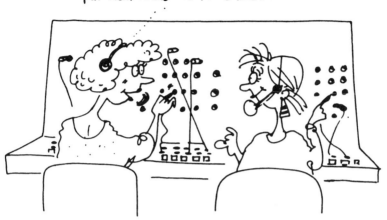

was wrong he said the ground was 'sour' around the tank because effluent had been seeping into the soil for so long it could no longer detoxify the waste matter.

Some people have stored so many negative emotions in their bodies for so long they have turned 'sour' like the soil around the septic tank. They are constantly unhappy, pessimistic and resistant to any advice. Whatever part of their body they 'go into' to retrieve a feeling they will discover a negative one. Whatever the bodily sensation they have it will turn out to represent a negative emotion.

With such people it is important to begin a long process of 'freshening the soil' and letting in some fresh air. By 'going into' the feelings, discovering their negative message and bringing it to conscious awareness, it is possible to reinvigorate them with some positive outlooks. If this is not done further 'sewage' is added to the overflowing containers and the 'bad smell' of negativity will be obvious to all those associated with such a person.

Use your feelings to help yourself by:

- acknowledging the feeling as a message – don't run away from it or remove it with a pill;
- 'going into' the feeling in a passive way – imagine you are inside the part of the body experiencing the feeling;
- 'sitting there' inside it and receiving any sensations – words you are telling yourself, pictures, memories, emotions. Convert the energy of the feeling into a message just as electricity can be converted into radio, TV, heat, or power;
- accepting the messages whatever they may be and however silly they seem, as genuine, helpful statements to provide you with knowledge;
- 'talking' to the messages as if they come from someone else, adding conscious knowledge and updating of information as well as acknowledging that the message has been received.

Two things will happen:

- the feeling will go away;
- you will understand what the feeling is all about and regard it in that light in future, not as a problem.

Rosanne has a fear of mice. It is an abnormal fear, a phobia. When she thinks of mice she gets a 'panic' feeling in her chest and her heart races. I asked her to create a little of that feeling while she was sitting opposite me. She was not too keen to do this as naturally she regarded the feeling as very unpleasant – something to be avoided.

She created a small part of the feeling in her chest by imagining a mouse. I then asked her to 'go inside' the feeling and receive any messages. After a few minutes she said she could hear herself telling herself to be more confident.

As she opened her eyes she smiled as that message was related to many other aspects of her life. In future, whenever she got that feeling, instead of regarding it as a *fear* or *phobia* she was going to remind herself to be *more confident* and not timid like the mice she feared.

Margaret works very hard in a factory. She and her supervisor are often at loggerheads. She has a weight problem and has been trying to lose weight for ages without much success.

When I asked her why she ate she said one of her main problems was at work when she felt very hungry and binged on sweets and cakes.

'How do you know you are hungry?' I asked. 'Because I get this hollow feeling in my tummy,' she replied, indicating a spot around her naval. 'Perhaps you are misinterpreting the feeling. I'd like you to learn a bit more about it. Just close your eyes and imagine you are inside that hollow feeling; notice any thoughts, words, pictures or emotions that are present there.'

After a few minutes she opened her eyes and exclaimed, 'It feels like anger, frustration, cheesed off due to work problems – I'm fed up, that's why I eat.'

We discussed alternative ways of dealing with the anger and frustration and decided she had a choice of (a) eating, (b) exploding, (c) telling the supervisor about it calmly or (d) making the opportunity to discuss the problem. She made a commitment to try one of these alternatives whenever the hollow feeling occurred and over the next month lost 12 pounds and only binged once.

Often people eat because of rumblings in their stomach; these noises are misinterpreted as hunger. This is completely incorrect because a small drink of water, which would have no effect on 'real' hunger, will stop the rumblings.

ANCHORING FEELINGS

We often recall memories when we see, hear or smell something that was associated with them. Walking past a baker's shop the smell of fresh bread may recall childhood memories of grandmother's baking. The good feeling and the smell have been 'anchored' together so that the emotion is reawakened by encountering the smell many years later.

We can use this phenomenon to our advantage by anchoring positive feelings in a way that will bring them into play when necessary. The following case history is a good example of how negative feelings can cause problems, whereas increasing positive feelings can bring benefits.

Bob felt depressed. He had felt low on many occasions over the last 10 years. He knew he was depressed by a tight feeling low down in his abdomen. When he felt that way he lost initiative and moped around, unable to enjoy or respond to his family's activities. He used alcohol to passify the feeling and usually went to bed inebriated hoping 'to sleep off' the depression.

Many factors in the past and present were involved in his problem and over a number of sessions he gained insight and more self-esteem but the depressed feeling remained. In order to see if we could minimize this negative feeling and perhaps increase any positive emotions in his possession, I asked him how he felt when he was successful in any way, whether in business, sport, love-making, singing etc.

He thought for a while, remembered a successful time in his life and smiled, placing his hand on the *top* part of his abdomen. 'When I feel good I have a tingling feeling here.

I remember when I kicked a winning goal playing soccer at school and I had that feeling then.'

'Good. I would like you to spend some time now gathering as many incidents as you can which have produced that feeling. Each time you remember an incident I want you to clasp your hands firmly together.' In this way I was attempting to 'anchor' the good feeling in his stomach with a voluntary clasping of his hands.

He sat quite still for about 15 minutes and every minute or so clasped his hands firmly together and then relaxed them. When he'd finished I talked to him about other things then asked him to clasp his hands as he had done before and he was pleasantly surprised when the positive feeling returned.

During the next week he spent time reinforcing his positive feeling and gradually learned to increase the time he felt that way by clasping his hands. Gradually, and with the help and encouragement of his family and friends, he felt his depressed feeling less often and an optimistic, confident feeling more often; he was able to alter the 'low' feeling to a 'high' one on many occasions and, by being much more in touch and in control of his feelings, was able to vary responses to daily situations.

'Anchoring' can be used in a variety of positive ways but, because of the direct link between the body and mind, we often anchor negative experiences without realizing it. Making use of this phenomenon to bring about positive results is essentially the same but requires persistence and guidance to ensure a permanent change.

For 'anchoring' to be successful it is essential to:

- create as many positive feelings as possible;
- each time one is remembered, 'anchor' it to a physical action in the present;

- 'trigger' the positive feeling by repeating the physical action.

PHANTOM LIMB TYPE FEELINGS

Someone who has lost a leg may develop a feeling of pain or itchiness in the foot that is no longer there. This is called 'phantom limb pain': it is very real and it gives us an incorrect message.

Many of our emotions are like this phantom limb pain. They are *real* feelings and are translated *incorrectly* by our minds. We feel the feelings and then unconsciously tell ourselves the feeling means 'X'. In fact, it may well be that the feeling is out of date and the interpretation 'X' is very misguiding.

Leah is 40 years old. She had an overpowering mother who continually blamed and badgered her throughout her childhood. She was terrified of doing anything wrong with anybody. If she went to tea and placed the teacup in a different position from its original place she got a feeling in her stomach telling her she was a bad person.

What was really happening was that she was getting a feeling in her stomach (due to her childhood upbringing) and was linking that to mean she was a bad person – because that was how her mother had brainwashed her.

In fact she was not a bad person. The interpretation of the feeling was completely incorrect and out of date.

The aim of therapy was to break the link between the feeling and Leah's interpretation of it. As this happened the feeling became less and less marked and she was able to feel less guilty and more balanced.

A book to help people with phobias is called *Feel The Fear And Do It Anyway*.

A sporting goods' company has it's slogan: 'Just do it.'

These statements are both aimed at reducing the mis-interpretation of feelings that direct and waylay us on our road to achievement.

EMOTIONS – PSYCHOLOGICAL FEELINGS

Emotions such as sadness, anger, fear and joy may or may not be accompanied by appropriate physical sensations. When asked how they know they feel angry, some people may describe a sensation in a part of their body or just a 'feeling in the mind' of being angry.

Difficulties arise when we fail to recognize or accept our emotions. The feeling is real, just as electricity is real. If we ignore it the consequences may be as disastrous as leaving a live wire lying around in the living room. Making the most of our emotions involves three stages:

- having the feeling;
- acknowledging the feeling;
- expressing the feeling.

Having the feeling In growing up we may have learnt to ignore some of our feelings or regard them as mad or bad and so may have lost touch with them. If a child feeling angry expresses that anger and receives a box over the ears, he or she may, like Pavlov's dogs, learn to ignore the feeling and interpret the feeling of anger as: anger = a box over the ears. So, not wanting to have a constantly ringing head, the child may choose to repress the feeling; in time access to anger becomes blocked off, and even when it would be appropriate it is unavailable.

When someone mentions they are feeling an emotion, say depressed, I often ask 'How do you know you are feeling depressed? Is it registered in some part of your body?' They may describe a heavy feeling on top of their head which occurs in certain situations. By going 'into this feeling' it may be possible to discover its origins, associated memories and the actual message intended. Often the analysis of the emotion releases a part of it and allows a calmness to replace it. The emotion may well be one from the past which is now inappropriate.

Alan wants to learn to swim. He is 30-year-old and misses a lot of fun with the family on holidays. He has attempted lessons on many occasions but a panicky feeling prevents him continuing with them.

When we discussed his panic he described it as a feeling of tightness in his chest and neck which was most unpleasant and directed him to 'run away'. As this seemed inappropriate for his lessons in the shallow training pool we decided to explore further. By going 'into' the 'panic' feeling in his chest a flood of memories surfaced, relating to incidents at school where the other boys laughed at him. As he was inept at many scholastic challenges he was the scapegoat of the class and had years of painful experiences where he wished he could 'run away' from everything.

His role with the swimming instructor reminded him so much of his school work that the associated feeling immediately returned. He also discovered that similar emotion-body sensations had prevented him learning to dance or drive. By 'talking' to this feeling and explaining 'things are different now, no-one will laugh, they are there to help and support', he was gradually able to allow courage and confidence to replace the out-of-date panic feeling that had restricted him for so long.

By analyzing the self-descriptions we have of ourselves

being sad, lonely, depressed, frightened and so on, we may discover 'new evidence' which could be helpful in freeing a restricted emotion imprisoned in the past for far too long.

Acknowledging the feeling Many people, because of their learning experiences, have access to certain feelings but deny them as wrong, often through a sense of guilt (see page 90). The emotion is felt and immediately followed by internal (or external) dialogue such as:

'I shouldn't feel that way';
'It's wrong to feel angry';
'I hate feeling lonely and so get drunk instead'.

It really is important that we learn to affirm, acknowledge and enjoy our feelings as a normal healthy part of ourselves. By doing so we remove the short-circuiting which is causing so much electrical damage to our bodies and minds. Accepting the feeling, owning it and not experiencing bad, mad, or guilty feelings about it, is a major step in the right direction *whatever the emotion is*.

Being able to feel angry, depressed, jealous, lustful, sad, greedy or lazy and tell ourselves that it is all right to have those feelings *for the time being*, allows their energy to flow rather than be held back like a pressure cooker. Acknowledging them does not mean we need to act on their behalf. Feeling angry and telling ourselves it is all right to feel angry does not mean we have to punch someone on the nose. We are affirming the emotions coming to our mind for a reason which may or may not be apparent. Verifying the feeling is like finding another piece in the jigsaw puzzle of being ourselves – a most important piece; indeed it might even be the 'missing peace'.

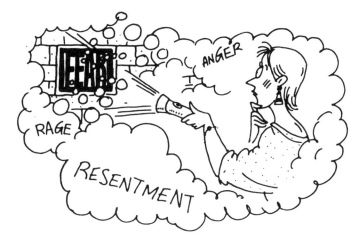

Expressing the feeling In order to restore internal calm it may be necessary to express the emotion you are feeling. It has built up and is 'looking for a way out'; if not acknowledged it may track in destructive directions seeking that outlet.

People with low self-esteem will often avoid expressing feelings for fear of hurting or upsetting someone (or themselves) as may have happened in childhood. It is not uncommon in therapy for an intense flood of emotions, stored for years, to be released with resulting peace and calm. Floods of tears not allowed earlier in life find their release in the safety of the therapist's understanding and support.

Learning to be more assertive allows a wider pathway for expressing feelings when they occur. But this learning may take a long time and require gentle support and guidance in order to build up the confidence that has been shattered by early experiences. Don't, however, make the quite common mistake of confusing 'assertive' with 'aggressive'; they are not related in any way. They are different emotions just as defence and attack are two forms of survival.

Allowing the emotion to be felt, acknowledged and flow on to expression creates self-confidence through personal experience in the present, rather than by relying on painful mislearning of the past. Many therapists believe that repressed feelings, such as anger, are causative factors in future illnesses – such as depression or hypertension. Expressing these feelings does not necessarily mean explosive outbursts but may be a suitable release of the acknowledged emotion.

In his excellent book *Focussing* (see page 229), Eugene Gendlin explains in simple terms how we can learn from our bodily sensations. He describes methods of listening to our bodies in receptive ways, acknowledging messages they have been trying to tell us for years. He comments: – 'Most people treat themselves very badly, much worse than they would ever think of treating another human being. Most people deal with their inside feeling person as a sadistic prison guard would.' Learning to alter this attitude to one of a compassionate friend brings about major positive changes.

A golfer carries a bag with a number of different clubs on a round of golf. These are constructed to deal with the different conditions on the golf course. A full set of clubs provides the golfer with choices according to the position of the ball. Our attitudes and feelings are similar to golf clubs – appropriate for some situations and inappropriate for others. By developing different attitudes and feelings and being able to acknowledge and express them, we will have greater confidence with which to deal with our lives. Imagine a golfer competing in a world-championship match with only two clubs and you will realize the emotional inadequacy we sometimes proffer to deal with situations that confront us. Just as it is not enough to own a fine set of clubs, so we must practise using our emotions and attitudes on 'the golf course of life' in order to become more proficient in living our lives.

It is important to remember that feelings and actions are separate entities. We can have a certain feeling, accept that feeling and yet act in a different way.

'I feel tired in the morning *so* I stay in bed';

'I feel tired in the morning *and* I get up to go to work', are two different ways of approaching a feeling. In the first case an inevitable linking is accepted; in the second the feeling and action are regarded as separate.

As we learn more about our emotions, understanding them and respecting them, we will come to live more in harmony with ourselves. We will be less controlled by our feelings and, at the same time, aim to control them less. After much patience, hard work and struggle, we may eventually be able to say 'I am feeling much better than before!'

Just as the clutch of a car can disconnect the engine from the wheel movement, so too can we separate feeling and action and thus, not be 'ruled' by our feelings but incorporate them into our total personality.

BALANCE

The concept of balance is a most important one when considering how we cope with life. When we feel bad, have psychological or physical problems, we could say we are out of balance.

There are many areas where balance applies. We can look at our diet, relaxation and exercise, the conscious and unconscious mind, work and leisure, logic and emotion.

If we consider a scale with logic at one end and emotion at the other, we could view people's characters as being either more logical or more emotional. The emotional person is run by his emotions while the logical one is bereft of them.

The aim is to have both logic and emotion – thoughts and feelings – balanced and in communication with each other. In this way we get the best of both worlds, and communication and relationships are easier and more successful.

One can tell when they meet a balanced person. There is a certain air about them which aids confidence and calmness for those around them. In a similar manner we can tell when someone is out of balance – they radiate tension, are all over the place or we just don't feel good in their presence.

John is an accountant. He works very hard and is success-ful in his job. He sees everything as black or white. He is unhappy and can't understand why. He has great difficulty with girlfriends: 'They just don't understand me.' He has great difficulties with colleagues: 'I just don't understand them.' He is completely out of touch with his emotions.

On the logical/emotional scales John is out of balance. His scales are heavily tipped on the direction of logic and he is out of depth when emotions (his or others) are involved.

His life is not what he expected and he has trouble understanding 'why it is not working'. He is too much in his head and not enough in his heart and the aim of therapy is to help restore this balance.

TURNING POINTS

1 Your feelings are important parts of every aspect of your life.
2 Learn to understand and translate correctly whatever feelings you find unpleasant.
3 'Going into' the feeling helps you to increase your knowledge of yourself.
4 Bringing 'up-to-date' information to a negative feeling may relieve it.
5 'Anchoring' is one way of putting positive feelings into the body.
6 Having the feeling, acknowledging and expressing it will prevent a build-up of limiting attitudes.
7 Decide where you are in the logic/emotional scale. Are you ruled by your head or your heart? Spend some time focusing on the weaker component learning how you can even up the scales a little.

PART 4

Analyzing the 'parts'

19

Analyzing the 'parts'

'In the land of the blind, the one-eyed man is king.'

'Every man has three characters – that which he exhibits, that which he has, and that which he thinks he has.'

'I can't go on', 'I'm always feeling insecure', 'I'm frightened of doing that' and similar comments are often heard in conversation. They are comments of resignation, of accepting an unacceptable situation, of having no control.

Such comments indicate (and create) a downward spiral, an inability to cope or a lowering of confidence. People holding such views have great difficulty in enjoying life to the extent that they might if they did not hold those beliefs.

One way out of being stuck in the quagmire of such self-limiting quotes is to view yourself as composed of different parts. This is an arbitrary formulation but has been very helpful in providing an avenue of escape. Len's case history will illustrate what I mean.

Len has a fear of leaving his home. He goes to work and

back but ensures that he is not delayed or diverted from his journey. He shops once a week and is in a state of constant anxiety until he gets home when he flops on the couch exhausted. He has tried many times to go out but panic sets in and he has to rush home. His friends have stopped inviting him anywhere and only occasionally drop in to see him.

He is miserable, would like to be free like other people but is resigned to the fact that he will possibly be a relative hermit for the rest of his life. He is overweight and doesn't look after himself, his hair is unkempt and clothes need repairing. A friend suggested to him that I might be able to help and he rang for an appointment.

Because of his problem he changed his appointment four times as he found it very difficult to fit in a visit to me in his extremely limited schedule of home – work – home. When he arrived he was very agitated and sat on the edge of the chair looking around the room and glancing at the clock. After he had explained his problem I pointed out that it appeared to me that there were two parts (at least) to Len. One wanted to be safe at home and one wanted to go out and be like everyone else. His nodding head indicated agreement.

I suggested that there was good reason for each part to believe the way it did, that perhaps in the past the housebound Len found security because of a situation that had occurred previously. He related how his early life was full of fears and anxieties, due to a neighbourhood gang which terrorized any schoolboy on the streets. Len ran the gauntlet each night on the way home from school and was badly beaten on a number of occasions.

As he grew older and left school, these beatings ceased, as the gang grew up and directed their attention towards more adult criminal behaviour. But the scared part of Len was not informed of this and so was always on the look out for trouble that had not occurred. As time went by and no attack took place this seemed to reinforce the frightened part's fear that it was inevitably just around the corner. In time these fears lost any relationship to the gang and just became a generalized fear.

All Len knew was that he felt anxious and frightened in any situation except home and work. Day after day, week after week, year after year, he reinforced this pattern and set in concrete the belief that this was the best (perhaps the only) way he could survive. When he tried to force himself to change, the protective part which had now been in control for years, took over and gave him a panic feeling. Sometimes when he went 'through' the panic feeling he felt free and revelled in that freedom all day. But the pain of 'going through' the fear was so great that he wasn't able to do this very often.

By learning to gradually communicate with the 'frightened part' and help 'it' feel less frightened by explaining that the gang had gone and it was now safe in the street, he began to see a ray of hope. I told him the story of the Japanese soldier who didn't know the war was over and remained in the jungle for years after armistice, fearful of being captured. Any attempts to convince him the war was over were construed as manoeuvres to capture him. He remained, living a life of fear and discomfort, for 30 years before eventually a document signed by the Emperor persuaded him to come out.

So it is with the frightened part. It needs careful and patient handling to allow it to 'come out of hiding'. It may be viewed as a frightened, suspicious part which needs an enormous amount of tolerance, understanding and support to let go of the pattern it has created. The false logic of this frightened part may be stated as follows: Len is going to be attacked by thugs. If I make sure he stays at home or goes to work he will be safe. I have forced him to do that for years and he is still alive and safe. Therefore my method is working and I must continue in order to protect him.

This logic is similar to the man on a London train who continually threw pink pieces of paper out of the window. When asked why he did this he replied, 'To keep away the wild elephants'. 'But there are no wild elephants here!' came the astounded reply. 'Effective isn't it!'

THE DANGERS OF CONFLICTING CUSTOMS

Part of us has one view of the world and how best to survive in it relating to previous experiences which have not been updated; opposing views may be held by the conscious part aware of present-day abilities but unaware of unconscious beliefs.

The continual battle between these two opponents who are unable to make contact, provides the energy to keep the problem going. Due to the inability to recognize each other's requirements there is a constant drainage of energy and self-confidence, a limitation to the power which would be available if the parts were working in the same direction.

By thinking of yourself as made up of parts, you can then change the part involved in the problem, rather than thinking it is the *whole of you* which should, but can't change.

I am not suggesting that this 'parts theory' represents the truth or facts; it is one method of achieving an understanding, a coping mechanism, a way of change. Some people are frightened they will be thought of as mad, a split personality or a schizophrenic if they 'talk to

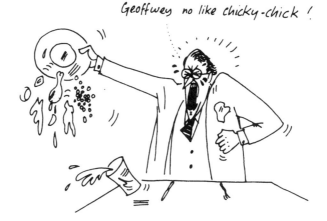

part of themselves'. What I believe is that this attitude is extending what we are already doing when we say, 'I'm in two minds about that' or 'I really want to speak up but I'm too frightened'. The suggestion I am making allows more control and understanding of our attitudes and behaviour.

An actress friend of mine suffering severe stage fright recognized the frightened part to be herself when she was very young. She created in her mind the frightened child and spent time every day talking to her. When she was in the dressing-room before a performance she would chat away to the 'little girl' explaining how nice it was to perform and there was nothing to fear. Her stage-fright disappeared and she looked forward to her acting with a much greater warmth and appreciation.

'Our emotions cause certain thoughts to arise in us. And these changing thoughts and desires cause a whole series of conflicting parts to come into existence.'
Gurdjieff

TURNING POINTS

1 You may find your problem easier to deal with by thinking 'part of me' is frightened, angry, lonely, guilty and so on.

2 Learn to communicate with that part via feelings, words, internal pictures.

3 Approach it with a caring, understanding, supporting attitude, not one of blame or anger.

4 Spend time each day with that part sharing your present-day knowledge.

5 You may be aware of the presence of the 'disturbed part' by uncomfortable feelings; acknowledge these feelings and communicate with them in a supportive and understanding way.

6 As the part becomes incorporated into your present life the uncomfortable feeling or symptom will become less.

20

The real me

> 'Any life, no matter how long and complex it may be, is
> made up of a single moment – the moment in which a man
> finds out, once and for all, who he is.'
> Jorge Luis Borges, Argentine writer

I hold a belief, unprovable, that inside each and everyone
of us is the 'real' person. This character has been influenced
by layers of experience, added as the years pass, to produce
the person they now are.

Often this present person is a distortion of the person
within. Parental influence, traumatic experiences,
repressed feelings all take their toll.

It is as if we are forced to play a part rather than being
ourselves. The saying 'To thine own self be true' has much
merit. The acting of a part created for us can be difficult,
painful and exhausting. If we can search and discover the
'real me' inside, life becomes so much easier.

'What if the real me is a rotter?' you may ask.

In my experience of seeing thousands of people over the
years, I believe the 'real me' is never a rotter. We are not

born troubled (although we may be negatively influenced by the birth process). The difficulties and restrictions in our present lives come from unsuitable teaching, blame, guilt and fear from not conforming to others' expectations.

One of the processes influencing our behaviour is 'a need to be loved' by others. However, when we convolute our personalities in order to be loved, we create more problems. As Andre Gide, the French writer, stated '*It is better to be hated for what you are than loved for what you are not.*'

This character 'the real me' is often sensitive, lacking in confidence and easily hurt. It needs support and encouragement but is often dismissed in order to portray the character required for the present.

WHO IS THE REAL ME?

How do we now who the real me character is?

The first step is to accept the concept of an inner person who is you. Once this has happened the energy for the discovery comes from awareness. Being aware how this inner person acts, what it needs, what its feelings are, will help you encourage it to become a greater part of yourself.

Some time after your acceptance of the inner personality you will find it speaking out for itself, requesting or demanding that its needs be fulfilled. You will become aware of things you really don't wish to do. You will learn to distinguish between doing what is best for you and doing things to please others. Many people are so frightened of being labelled as *selfish* they ignore the 'inner me' altogether.

You will know when the you and the 'inner me' come close together because you will feel good. Doubts and conflicts will lessen. You will be more sure of yourself and what is right for you in spite of others' comments. You will feel happier spending time by yourself rather than seeking others' approval. In time the 'real me' will grow and integrate with you to become one and the same.

As you get closer to being yourself there will be less 'shoulds, ought to's and musts' occurring in your thoughts and speech. These will be replaced by 'wish to, going to, decided to' which means you are owning your power.

This process is not an easy one. There are many pressures for us to perform in a manner foreign to our real desires. Criticism and blame force us to back into a previous role. However difficult the journey is, the end result is certainly worthwhile.

TURNING POINTS

1   Describe to yourself the 'real me' inside.
2   How does he/she differ from yourself?
3   In what areas are there conflicts of choice atti-
    tude, behaviour between you and the 'real me'?
4   Set yourself daily tasks to learn more about who
    you really are and take risks to act and behave
    that way in spite of any critical comments you
    may receive.

21

The memory lingers on

'Like the wars and winters
Missing behind the windows
Of an opaque childhood.'
Philip Larkin, *Forget What Did*

'Beware lest you do not lose the substance by grasping at
the shadow.'
Aesop

How often do we get good or bad feelings, not from what
is happening, but from an association with past events?
The smell of freshly roasted coffee reminded us, perhaps of
meals with friends or a holiday abroad and we continue on
our way with an inner smile. The sensation of smell has
triggered off a 'search' in the back of our mind for a similar
experience. When this experience is remembered an associated feeling occurs. Often the memory is not brought to
the conscious mind and we just 'feel good' without
knowing why.

Mrs Johnson sat down in front of me smiling. 'How are you today doctor?' she enquired politely. 'I'm fine thank you' I replied. 'How were things last week?' She immediately burst into tears, as she recollected the calamities which had befallen her during the previous week. The fact that they were mostly resolved and not an immediate problem indicated that it was the memories from the past that were causing her to feel unwell in the present.

'Why discuss memories when there is nothing you can do about them?' you may be asking. In fact it *is* possible to alter them and provide yourself with a positive rather than a negative guide to your behaviour. To change your memories may seem preposterous but I can assure you it is possible, simple and effective.

Imagine that your memories are stored in an immense room in the back of your mind with a door to your conscious mind in front. Either spontaneously (as with the smell of coffee) or as a result of reflection (as with Mrs Johnson), you can achieve recall of past experiences. This back room contains memories from birth – some would even say before birth – recorded and stored in different ways.

Imagine the walls of the room lined with books – thousands of books, all different sizes and shapes, bindings and colours; printed in a variety of characters and boldness, some large with illuminated lettering, others small and barely decipherable. On other walls films are being shown. These too are in a variety of sizes and colours. Some are small, like TV films, others are cinemascope, still others are black and white. Tape recordings playing in another part of the room convey messages, speeches, sounds of events, music, parents' voices.

Your conscious mind has a remarkably specific way of

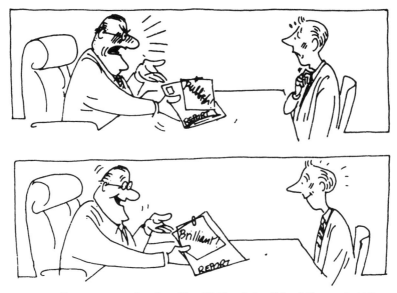

IT IS POSSIBLE TO ALTER MEMORIES AND PROVIDE YOURSELF
WITH A POSITIVE RATHER THAN A NEGATIVE GUIDE TO YOUR
BEHAVIOUR

choosing from the storeroom of memories. At different
times, due to different situations, a certain memory will
become more prominent and affect the present feeling.
Some memories are much more profound and recur continually in the conscious mind. These may be times of fear,
pain, disaster, guilt, sadness. Someone whose early life had
an abundance of these experiences may often be flooded by
unpleasant thoughts triggered by something that was seen,
said or heard in the present.

'I can't understand it doctor. I have a lovely home and
husband, my children are happy and healthy, I have no
reason to feel sad yet I am constantly crying.' This may be
a statement from someone who is having unpleasant
memories continually thrust through the door into the
conscious mind.

CHANGING MEMORIES

One way of helping improve the situation is to change unpleasant memories. In reality what we are storing is *our opinion* of what happened a long time ago. Anyone who has heard witnesses giving evidence in a trial will understand how the truth can be distorted quite unintentionally. Five witnesses to a car accident may all believe they are telling the truth but give five completely different versions of what happened. The more time that has elapsed since the accident, the more varied will be the accounts of it.

You may say, 'But I know my memory is accurate because it happened to *me*, I didn't see it happen to someone else'. That is quite true, but the distance of time may well have distorted the image as well as the state of mind you were in at the time of the incident.

If, as a child, Bob was pushed under the water while swimming and thought he would drown, such an intense experience would be recorded in the 'back room' with great prominence, so that any associated action – going swimming, for example – would bring that panicky feeling forward to the present. Bob is now 30 and by viewing that experience from the present he could allow it to assume a proportionate representation in his mind. It was a time of a few seconds – which seemed like hours – when due to a lark he thought he would drown. He may be able to look at it and laugh and add associated thoughts and ideas which would allow him to feel comfortable with the memory. He may dilute it with the passage of time that has occurred, so instead of it being a cinemascope film with loud stereo sound, it may become a small black-and-white TV film playing softly. By making such changes the impact of this distant event on his present-day life would be reduced and he could enjoy his life unmarred by that memory. He could go swimming and even put his head under the water without feeling his previous panic.

When people come to see me and say, 'I feel depressed, unhappy, guilty, lonely', I may ask them, 'How did you learn to feel this way?' We then track back through their experiences to find how they learned to have that feeling, how it became part of their repeated way of experiencing life.

It is important to take the past out of the present. Memory changing involves six simple steps:

- remember an incident in the past which causes discomfort when you recall it;
- go through the incident from beginning to end as if it is a film you are watching. Note any associated feelings;
- run through the film again and stop (freeze) one frame which represents the incident best and has the associated negative feeling incorporated in it;
- allow a frame – a picture frame – to surround this still picture;
- change the picture any way you like in order to make it pleasant, humorous, light-hearted, happy or positive. You have free artistic licence to do anything you wish to achieve this and notice if the frame changes too;
- stay looking at the changed picture, having associated good feelings and rubbing out the old one.

You are probably saying this is all too easy, it won't work, memories are fixed and unchangeable. This is not so. What happens in the mind is that an event is fixed in place, with the intensity with which it occurred. It may remain at that intensity even though years of positive living should have diluted it and reduced its prominence. Many other incidents have occurred which could allow the person to put a completely different perspective on the event, but they are not allowed to do so because the mind has 'walled off' the memory. Going through the steps above brings the memory out into the light of our present-day abilities and viewpoints and changes it to a more appropriate and helpful nature.

Sybil had had chronic neck and back pain for eight years following a fall. She had received many treatments and her attitude was a mixture of pain, anger, sadness, hopelessness and frustration.

She recalled the many treatments when her pain was increased and there was associated anger at the uncaring attitude of the doctors. I suggested we change some of those memories as they were not helping her in her present plight. She recalled the mixture of fear, anger and frustration at the thought of the week-long traction she was involved in at the start of her treatment.

In her mind she ran through the film of the traction experience and changed it to one where she removed the traction apparatus and stormed out of the hospital screaming abuse at all the staff. In another incident, with a painful and ineffective neck collar, she altered the picture to one where the surgeon was encased in a similar painful collar and she became the therapist, telling him in an off-hand manner to wear the collar for one month.

The aim of memory changing is to alter a negative or painful recollection into a positive, humorous or pleasant one. The ways in which this is done depend entirely on the creativity of the person concerned. Patients with an open attitude and vivid imagination use this technique to great advantage. Those with fixed ideas find it very difficult to comprehend a concept of changing past representations.

It is also possible to make use of 'future memories'. If a recurring event produces unpleasant feelings, it may be feasible to imagine that future event associated with positive feelings.

Tom hated making after-dinner speeches. He was not confident at the best of times. Three years ago he had been stuck for words and the speech was a disaster. He couldn't possibly imagine that scene changed and he was due to give another speech in three weeks' time.

I asked him to create a 'future memory' which he felt comfortable with. After some discussion he found a picture of himself talking, supported by the friendly (slightly inebriated) audience who were unaffected by the quality of his speech.

This picture allowed him to feel comfortable, confident and relaxed; he looked at it in his mind twice a day for the next three weeks and also just before he got up to speak. It went well; he couldn't remember anything about the speech but everyone seemed reasonably happy and he didn't have that terrible tense feeling associated with his previous speeches.

It is true that a picture is worth a thousand words and pictures instilled in the back of the mind will override any conscious encouragement either from outside or inside. Perhaps it is time to change some of the pictures in your gallery, so they may help rather than hinder your life in the present. In doing so you may be able to say to yourself 'Thanks for the memory'.

'The truth you speak
Has no past and no future . . .
It is
And that's all it needs to be.'
Richard Bach, *Illusions*

TURNING POINTS

1 Ask yourself what role negative memories are playing in your present attitudes or feelings.
2 Choose a single unhappy memory that creates negative feelings.
3 Go through the six steps described earlier and alter the memory to a positive one with its associated pleasant feelings.
4 Choose a 'future memory' which has associated fears or doubts.
5 Change the 'future memory' by the six steps into one with a positive outcome.
6 Each day make a commitment to change a negative memory into a positive one.

22

Creative visualization

Our minds work on many levels (see Chapter 13). One of these levels is a world made up of pictures. It is not imagination as the world is 'real' and does not come from our trying to create it. Similarly, our dreams are real when we are in them; they have a life of their own – so does this world I am talking about.

You may ask why such a phenomenon appears in a self-help book. Surely, you may say, we all know about childish fantasy, but that has no real bearing in the world of problems and experience.

You would be quite wrong to come to that conclusion. Learning about these pictures and becoming involved in the process of creative visualization can cause marked, profound and lasting changes to your life.

The aim is to learn about your inner world through the pictures, not pictures you consciously create but those that are already there to be discovered. As you go 'inside' you can translate feelings into pictures. This is done passively by allowing things to develop and following the pictures where they lead you.

Josephine had been having feelings of tension in her neck and shoulders for months. Her sleep was disturbed; she was irritable and unhappy. She knew something was wrong but she was unable to deal with it.

I asked her to close her eyes and relax for a minute or two. I suggested she moved from the 'trying' attitude to the passive 'being' state of mind. I next asked her to 'go inside' and focus on her neck and shoulders from within. After a minute of silence I asked her what she could see in there.

'I can see two groups of little men in strange outfits having a tug of war with a rope in my neck.'

I said; 'What would you like to do about that?'

After half a minute's silence she slowly replied; 'I'd like to ask them to stop as it's hurting me.'

I suggested she do just that and she sat for the next few minutes in silence concentrating intently on what was occurring in her mind.

'What is happening now, Josephine?' I asked quietly.

'The men are not pulling so hard, the rope is slackening.'

'Why don't you talk to the men for a few minutes and find out how they came to be there and what are their aims?'

Again intense silence. Tears started to well up in her eyes and roll down her cheeks.

'They said they have been trying to help me, they belong to two groups with different ideas. One group wants me to be assertive the other thinks I'll be happier if I'm passive and don't cause any problems.'

'Let them know you will spend time with them from now on so you can all work together. Tell them you want to understand them and not have them in conflict.'

After a few more minutes' silence Josephine opened her eyes, wiped away her tears and drowsily said: 'That was very strange. Am I going mad talking to little men in my shoulder?'

She burst into laughter from relief and fatigue from the process she had been involved in.

'No Josephine, you are not going mad. In fact in my opinion you are going sane,' and we both laughed together.

Josephine's past history has been one of conflict with herself and her parents. She received different messages from them about being assertive and also avoiding confrontation. The men in her neck were pictorial representatives of that conflict and she used this symbolism to resolve this problem and remove the painful tension.

VISUALIZATION WITH CHILDREN

Because the child's world is so full of imagery they respond to this technique very easily and quickly. It is an ideal method of resolving children's problems because it is fun, simple and fits in with their understanding of life.

The child's inner world is full of mystical figures – dragons, dwarfs, witches, caverns, tunnels and colours. As we grow and adults tell us 'stop day-dreaming; don't be silly, that's not real' we lose contact with this world.

Anne, aged 10, had been through troubled times when her parents divorced. In four years the tension had been reflected by screwing up her toes in her shoes. This led to callouses which caused her pain and concern.

As she described it:

'My toes feel itchy. I screw them up against the end of my shoes which stops the itch for a few seconds, then I relax them and they itch again. This goes on all day and only stops when I go to sleep at night.'

I asked her to 'go inside' and look at the mechanism involved. With gentle guidance she saw nerves taking itchy messages from her toes to her mind. These were coloured red; other green nerves were coming from her mind to her toes telling them to screw up.

Between us we worked out a way of blocking the green messages so the itchy message had no return vehicle to complete the habit circuit.

Almost immediately Anne was able to leave her toes at rest for a few minutes – something she had been unable to do for four years. I made a tape for her so she could repeat the blocking of the 'screwing' message each day.

In two weeks the habit had been reduced by 80 per cent and in a month had gone altogether. Anne was delighted by the adventure, so was her Dad who sat in during the session.

Lucy is a bright 11-year-old. She had been operated on six times by the time she was four. She has (understandably) an extreme phobia of doctors, nurses, hospitals and blood.

Her mother Diana has a warm and close relationship with Lucy and has tried many things to reduce her fear. She talked with Lucy, played doctors and nurses, explained what had happened, but Lucy's fears remained uncontrollable.

Diana heard of the visualization technique and came to see me about it. She did not bring Lucy in case it would increase her fears. We talked about the previous operations, hospital treatment, blood transfusions and all the experiences that combined to make Lucy so frightened.

I explained visualization and demonstrated it with Diana so she had the experience of knowing what I was talking about. I explained that it should be used gently and with respect to Lucy's responses.

Three weeks after Diana's visit I received an excited phone call to tell me the news. Diana had gradually introduced 'the picture game' at bed time. Lucy had become excited and asked to play it each night. When she 'went inside' to explore her fear she found a large wolf with a long wound on his stomach that was oozing blood.

Lucy was terrified of the wolf and with Diana's patient help she learnt to tentatively stroke it. The wolf became friendly and licked her. As the nights passed the oozing stopped and the wound started to heal.

Over the three weeks Diana detected a minor change in Lucy's attitude towards blood. She seemed less frightened and became more confident in herself. It was early days but Diana knew things were improving.

Over the following months Lucy and the wolf became firm friends. The wolf protected her and she shared all her secrets with him. The wolf's wound healed completely and Lucy's fear of blood decreased to be a fraction of what it previously was. One day she scratched her leg and instead of making a scene just asked for a band aid. She spent a long time with her friend the wolf that night.

Diana told me how delighted she was with the whole exercise. She commented that it was fun, Lucy enjoyed it, no white-coated doctors had been involved and Lucy had the feeling she had cured herself.

The technique can be adopted to help many childhood difficulties – fear, aches and pains, school phobias, bed wetting, nightmares, shyness etc. It requires a 'facilitator' – someone who supports the child in the exploration of the inner world. This could be the parent or therapist who is supporting, caring and uses 'clean language' so as not to impose beliefs of their own.

HOW DOES IT WORK?

1 The person wishing to learn about feelings etc., sits quietly with eyes closed.
2 The facilitator gently and slowly guides them to go inside and focus on the part of the body where the feeling is.
3 Allowing time for exploration the person relates what is seen. No logical assessment or judgment is allowed to dilute the experience.
4 The pictures are allowed to have their own form and may relate to past experiences or memories.
5 Whatever occurs in the picture is respected and treated as real.
6 The person can talk to any animal or person who occurs in the picture to learn why they are there, when they started and what they are trying to achieve.
7 The process may continue for ten to twenty minutes and be repeated on a daily basis so a pattern will be seen to evolve.

TURNING POINTS
1 Choose a feeling or emotion which is causing you trouble, limiting you.
2 Make some time to explore it using the techniques described.
3 Allow the feeling to be converted into pictures; alter the pictures if you choose so that the reciprocal feeling is improved, e.g. if guilt is represented as black change it to a rosy colour.

23

The forgotten child within

Our actions and attitudes can be affected by the child within. When this internal person feels at ease and comfortable our life is so much easier.

We are all affected by how our parents treat us. I am not in any way blaming parents but pointing out that our childhood experiences play a major role in how we turn out as adults.

Often when we lack confidence, develop fears, have difficulties, it is as if the child within us is affecting our behaviour. One aim of growing up, becoming an adult, is to have the inner child integrated so we make choices from an adult perspective.

Probably the most powerful and emotional technique I use I call 'helping the forgotten child within'. This involves becoming a parent to ourselves. It releases many vivid emotions and allows out-of-date behaviour to be resolved.

Imagine parents who restrict their child with blame, guilt, fear or non-acceptance. This child may well have problems in adulthood because its potential has not been encouraged and nurtured. Limitations in self-esteem, doubt and lack of confidence all cause difficulties and restrictions.

The technique I use is to act as a facilitator to the person opposite me, encouraging them to be supportive, understanding, caring parents to their child within. This involves relaxation, visualization, getting in touch with buried memories and release of pent up emotion.

Another way of looking at it is as if we are viewing a film. The film is our life story. In childhood some of the frames are frozen and the child in those pictures doesn't grow as the film progresses. That child remains in the state of fear, guilt, helplessness or shyness and continues to influence us unless released from the frozen frame.

Tina is a 36-year-old artist, married with two children. Outwardly she is successful, confident and contented. She disclosed to me that this was all a mask. Inside she is fearful, nervous and unable to make decisions.

Tina's childhood was one of uncertainty due to an alcoholic mother. When Tina came home from school she never knew what to expect. Some days she was greeted by a caring mother full of love and warmth. Other days she returned to find a dishevelled, drunken figure in nightdress roaming around the house muttering incoherently to herself. Tina learnt never to bring schoolfriends home in case it was one of mother's 'bad days'. She learnt to steel herself as she opened the door and gradually formed an outer façade to deal with the facts. She was often terrified of finding her mother dead, or of being abused or abandoned.

Tina's father left home when she was 14 and this triggered off a change in her mother. She went to AA, and after a period of time stopped drinking altogether, becoming the warm mother Tina had seen glimpses of previously.

When she was 22 Tina met Graham. They were married and for the last 14 years have had a stable and happy marriage bringing up their two lovely daughters. Tina is very happy in her present situation but those years of early childhood still haunt her and diminish her ability to enjoy all the benefits she now has. Her mother is still alive and well, and once a month Tina and her family visit her for Sunday lunch.

I explained to Tina the concept of the forgotten child within. She acknowledged that it was applicable to her and agreed to work helping the young Tina.

I asked her to close her eyes, focus on her breathing, relax and move from the 'trying' mode to the 'being' mode. When she was ready I asked to allow a picture of the young Tina to appear in her mind.

After a minute or two she burst into tears and described a little girl aged 5 whose life was haunted by the fear that her mother may die due to her drinking. I allowed her to cry for a minute or two before asking:

'And did her mother die?'

'No she didn't', she slowly whispered through her tears.

'Well why don't you let the little girl know her mother doesn't die, in fact she gets better and is still alive and well 30 years later.'

Tina was silent for a few minutes, intent on her internal dialogue with the terrified little girl inside, helping by updating her and telling her about her mother and the good changes that happen in her life.

'How did the little girl respond?' I gently questioned.

'She is very cautious and doesn't really believe me.'

'That's right. That's how we are when we are frightened. I'd like you to spend time with her over the next week, being her friend, listening to her and helping her.'

Tina went away and spent time over the following weeks

with the 'child within'. The child became less scared and Tina's confidence grew as result. It took many months and lots of ups and downs, but eventually the child within became integrated and Tina's fears, doubts and indecision improved in the process.

Getting in touch with the child within, helping it in a caring and supportive way reveals many emotions, attitudes and memories. The process of resolving these helps us a great deal in becoming adults, feeling good about ourselves, taking responsibilities and dealing with life's problems in a more balanced way.

TURNING POINTS

1 Consider some of your actions, attitudes or emotions as if they are coming from the child within.
2 Spend some quiet time getting in touch with this inner child by visualization, talking to it or being aware of its feelings.
3 When communicating with this child help in a supportive way just as you would help a child of your own. Allow it to express its feelings without blame or guilt.
4 Notice how the child within changes with time.

24

Panning for gold

As you go through life make this your goal – keep your eye
upon the doughnut and not upon the hole
Sign in a doughnut cafe

Of all the techniques I use to help people overcome their
problems the one I call 'Panning for Gold' has the most
success in the shortest amount of time. A number of
patients have remarked how they have made positive
changes after only a few weeks of using this technique.

An affirmation is a saying which when repeated achieves
positive results. If you repeat to yourself 'I feel great and
I'm a very confident person', in time this has the desired
effect.

When I tried to use affirmations a voice in my head kept
saying:

'That is all rubbish, you are trying to fool yourself, it is
not so,' and the affirmation had no effect. Because of this
I created the 'Panning for Gold' concept where we use *our
own* experiences as the affirmations.

It is a fact that many people focus on the negative aspects

of their lives – things that may go wrong, failures that have occurred, critical comments received. This focus on the negative is habit forming and contagious. After a while your gatherings and discussions drift towards doom and gloom.

Joe is a hardworking businessman. He has real worries and imaginary worries. He also has successes in all areas of his life. He is not happy, his wife is not happy and even his children are beginning to be unhappy.

When I talked to him about how his mind worked, what his attitude was, he replied that he always focused on mistakes that had happened, or might happen in order to deal with or prevent them.

When he came home and his wife asked how his day went he always brought up negative things that had happened. They would spend the rest of the evening discussing these and becoming more and more involved with disappointments and failures. When he went to sleep he tossed and turned wrestling with failures past and future.

In general Joe was turning his head to face negativity and becoming absorbed by it in the process.

I suggested he spend some time before going to sleep focusing on the good things that had happened that day. I told him there were obviously going to be negative things that had happened but this exercise was to ignore them and focus on the good things however small.

Three weeks later Joe returned saying he felt so much better. The exercises were difficult at first but now had become routine. He had discussed our consultation with his wife and both agreed to talk mainly about good things when he came home.

And so 'Panning for Gold' was born.

The metaphor is of a gold prospector looking for gold in

his pan as he swills the water over the gravel and mud in it. He knows there is a lot of dirt there but he doesn't focus on it. His eye is alert for the glitter from the speck of gold.

'Panning for Gold' is very useful for people with low self-esteem, lack of confidence, improving attitudes, in fact for most people.

The exercise consists of spending ten minutes or so before you go to sleep to re-live your day. Start from when you woke up and go through the day slowly noticing the good things that have happened. Pass over and ignore things that were not positive.

Good experiences (specks of gold) come in all forms from the very minor:

'Gee that shower was lovely when I woke up'
'I saw a mother gazing lovingly into her baby's eyes'
'I was so relieved to catch that bus I thought I'd missed'

to the larger nuggets:

'My boss said I may be in line for a promotion'
'I did something really assertive today when I answered back to that rude cashier at the supermarket.'

As the gold prospector grows wealthy by adding grain after grain of gold to their purse, so reviewing your day in a positive light has the same effect. The added bonus is that when you go to sleep your thoughts are in a positive direction and your unconscious responses – dreams – follow in a similar vein, giving you eight hours benefit from the ten minute exercise.

TURNING POINTS

1   Compare your present attitude to the gold pros-
    pector. Are you focusing on the gold specks or the
    dirt?

2   Before going to sleep at night examine the day
    focusing on the pleasant experiences you have
    had.

3   Allow good feelings, self praise to result from
    these reflections.

4   Stay focused on those positive feelings and experi-
    ences as you drift off to sleep.

25

Alternative choices

'You can choose any colour you like as long as it is black.'
Henry Ford

'The best-laid schemes o' mice an' men
Gang aft a-gley (awry)
An' lea'e us nought but grief an pain
For promis'd joy!'
Robert Burns, *To a Mouse*

In long-term problems many solutions are available, some more acceptable than others. One aim may be to be in a position to choose from the alternatives; once in that position the next step is to take responsibility for the pathway chosen.

Studying available choices more closely it often becomes apparent that many people are imprisoned by the *illusion of choices*; that is they feel they are free to go in different directions but in fact are limited, either internally or externally, to the routes available to them.

'I could give up smoking if I wanted to.'
'I will ask the boss for a rise when the time is appropriate.'

These are comments with an underlying belief that these actions are possible. In fact due to limitations they may *not* be possible and the anticipated choices are unavailable.

In order to be free to chose we need:

- to know what to do,
- to know how to do it;
- to believe we are capable of doing it;
- to make a commitment to do it.

It may well be that any solution to a long-term problem requires us to change our behaviour; thus availing ourselves of a new choice, a new direction, a different attitude. But because of the debilitating nature of chronic problems

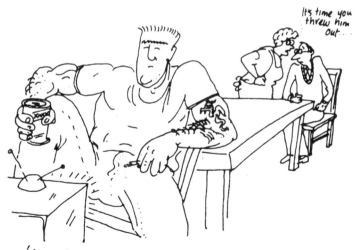

'IN ORDER TO TRY SOMETHING NEW WE NEED IMPROBABILITY OF FAILURE ...'

we are extremely wary of any new venture outside the safety of our experience. Just as a man sinking in quicksand soon realizes that every attempt to extricate himself causes him to sink further, so the chronic sufferer learns to *avoid* choices in case they make things worse rather than better.

In order to try something new we need time, support and encouragement, a logical explanation about the possibilities of success (and improbability of failure), courage and the knowledge of what to do and how to do it. The choices offered need to be acceptable to our abilities and outlook. It is no use advising a wife to be stronger with her husband if she is unable to because of previous damaging experiences caused by a strong parent. The advice may be correct, but as the 'how to do it' is missing there is, in reality, no new choice.

A list of some 'helpful hints' may provide an understanding of your position:

- we do the best we can with the choices available;
- increasing your choices is one way of improving your situation;
- you often create your own limitations and so reduce the number of choices available;
- if what you are doing is not working try something different;
- alter your attitude to your problem, viewing it positively;
- symptoms are often messages about psychological needs;
- stress and tension drain energy and prevent the use of your natural resources;
- problems are often maintained by the restrictions of fear and guilt;
- spending time on yourself daily is a basic requirement

for body and mind;
- learning to accept yourself, like yourself, gain self-confidence, is a major aim in life;
- many improvements occur by 'facing up' to things rather than avoiding them;
- time and effort are two major requirements for change;
- being flexible allows a greater opportunity to benefit from situations and relationships;
- 'concrete facts' often turn out to be 'fixed attitudes'.

There are two further points to add to this list:

- try not to try too hard to resolve your problem;
- try to remember the beneficial effects of humour.

I agree that both points may well come into the 'easier said than done' category, but give them a try, they can work out.

Ed was a keen amateur cricketer. He had done so well as a batsman in the second team of his club that he had been promoted to the first eleven. But then things started to go wrong. He was trying so hard to make good scores that he was generally out before he had made 10 runs.

With some difficulty, I persuaded him to stop trying to make any runs at all – to stay in, but not to score.

When I saw him next he was very shamefaced and apologetic.

'I'm very sorry I didn't follow our agreement', he said.

'What happened?' I replied, annoyed.

'Well, I went in to bat and did just as you said. I made sure I didn't make any runs but when we adjourned for lunch I was 56. I continued trying not to score and just before stumps I was 92. I remember in the last over people shouting from the boundary to hit out as we needed two to win. I persisted in blocking but unfortunately smacked a boundary on the third last ball.'

'Life is not a carnival, it's a damned circus.'

Remember, *humour* is a very powerful ingredient in improving situations. It may be that people have a better sense of humour when they are feeling well or that one feels better when something humorous occurs. It would certainly seem appropriate, if it were possible, to bottle and sell fun on prescription as a remedy for most disorders. The positive energy liberated by laughter has been known for ages. Having a more lighthearted attitude is certainly more suitable for recovery than the heavy, gloomy one which naturally accompanies chronic illness.

The power of laughter was described by Norman Cousins in his book *Anatomy of an Illness*. He was suffering from a painful and disabling condition of his muscles and had difficulty in walking. His doctors predicted a long and crippling disease, possibly resulting in death. After intensive hospital treatment he decided to leave hospital, book into a hotel and try a therapy of vitamin C and laughter. He hired a number of comedy films including the Marx Brothers and laughed all day. Over a period of time, his symptoms abated and his disease resolved itself. His laughter provided a cure in a situation where medicine had failed. Often such an alternative approach to a problem can provide a solution, where 'more of the same' – trying harder and longer – fails or augments the trouble.

So, one way of approaching a problem is to analyze all the components involved in trying to *solve* it. As these are obviously not succeeding (or the problem would not persist), it is worthwhile providing alternatives for each

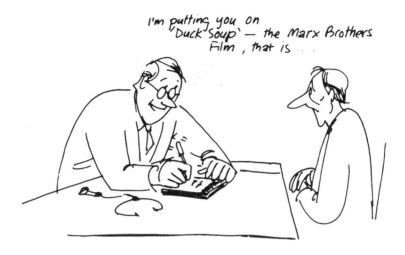

HUMOUR IS A VERY POWERFUL INGREDIENT

component and observing the result of trying them. But here again we can run into trouble as this example shows:

Research workers had noticed how cow dung was used as fuel by the poor in rural India, and set about to devise a simple and efficient stove to improve their quality of life. The researchers produced a remarkably effective stove, and it was introduced into the countryside as an example of the benefits of modern science for the world's poor. But the outcome was the reverse of the expected improvement. Rich people noticed how effective the stoves were and sent their servants to collect all the dung available, and the poor ended up worse off than before.

This case suggests that while looking for a solution, it may be advisable to be aware of the benefits of the present predicament and query how you may be worse off if that problem is solved. A problem may often be a solution of sorts, as suggested by John Harrison in his book *Love Your Disease, it's keeping you healthy*.

When taking the responsibility for a change in your situation choose a very small part of the problem you wish to alter, don't attempt anything too mammoth or disappointment will inevitably ensue. Realize that the more you learn about the problem the more understanding you will have about yourself, so that the solution really will be a solution and not one more false trail or red herring.

TURNING POINTS

1 Recognize that the situation you are in offers more than one choice for your actions and attitudes.

2 Make a list of possible choices available and what is preventing you attempting them.

3 Examine your limitations to see if they are due to external factors or internal attitudes.

4 Check on the points listed in the chapter and apply them to your problem.

5 It may well be that 'trying to change' is preventing change.

6 Make an effort to add humour to your life.

26

Taking responsibility

'Symptoms are potentially meaningful and purposeful conditions.'
Arnold Mindell, *Working With the Dreaming Body*

'A man should not strive to eliminate his complexes but to get into accord with them.'
Sigmund Freud

How can one write about a solution to a continuously existing problem? Some readers of this book will have hoped that it would supply all the answers – simply, quickly and efficiently; unfortunately that is not the case. Chronic problems generally persist because that road has already been tried and failed. In spite of loud laments many problems are maintained by trying short cuts, wasting energy unnecessarily, not taking responsibility, misinterpreting messages and the many other cogs in the carousel.

A book is a book, it is not a solution but consists of ideas and thoughts from one person's point of view – mine. Some of these messages may be more helpful than others – that is they are more obviously appropriate to your specific problem. Other suggestions may provide a basis for future learning.

There are many metaphors about struggles to overcome difficulties – fables, nursery tales and folklore abound in them. The game of chess provides many ingredients that are useful comparisons to the battles we play in our own personal lives. The components of significance are: the opponent, aim of the game, strategies employed, values of the individual pieces, moves available and the end result. The game requires patience, effort, wisdom, understanding and an ability to vary the approach depending on the situation. It is also important to understand your opponent, his or her attitudes and methods, and to plan ahead allowing time to create patterns and plans which may involve a fluctuation of strengths. At times it is necessary to sacrifice a piece to make a gain; at other times a defensive move may prove to be the most attacking one. Just when you feel you have won, you discover you have lost, and vice versa.

Playing against an experienced opponent (as` chronic problems certainly are) it is essential to know the rules and value of each piece in the game. Being unaware of the potential of certain pieces in certain situations means you are not achieving the most from your game. If, in losing a game, you learn – then you have won, as there will be many more games ahead of you. The unseen rules concerning patience, anticipation, lateral thinking, respect for your partner, all play as vital a role in your life as on the chessboard.

Changing an attitude often solves the problem. This was delightfully illustrated in a story told by the famous American psychiatrist Dr Milton Erickson:

As a teenager he was brought up on a farm. One day a new bull was delivered, and his father needed to house it in a shed. It was facing the shed and 10 paces away but strongly resisted any attempts to pull it forward.

His father struggled, sweated and cursed as he tugged on the rope attached to the ring through the bull's nose; young Milton sat in the shade occasionally commenting *he* could get the bull into the shed. His father ignored these comments until the sun was setting and the beast had not budged one inch.

'OK smart boy, show me how to do it' said the exasperated father.

Milton calmly walked behind the bull, grabbed his tail with both hands and pulled with all his might. The startled animal took a step towards the shed. This procedure was repeated until the bull was safely housed in the shed and his bewildered father left scratching his forehead.

In the quest for a solution, the one unknown factor is *time*. No-one can accurately predict when a chronic problem will be resolved; the many frustrations and disappointments due to repeated failures cause a great drain of energy. But the pattern of long-term problems makes it essential that no eager, rapid predictions are made as they may lead to another disappointment and further entrenchment of the problem. Many people will fall by the wayside of avoidance, despondency and hopelessness, and will continue in their circular tracks, losing sight of any hope ahead.

Taking responsibility means accepting the problem as *yours*, and that you will do everything in your power to deal with it. This often means going against advice from those who 'should' know. (It is not uncommon for members of the medical profession to claim 'we doctors know what's right, and any alternative would be foolish'.) But there is no panacea available, no swift easy solutions, each journey is as unique as its owner's fingerprints. There are so many useful words of advice, hints, techniques which may help you on your way, or point out repeated dead ends. In the long run it is up to you to make the most of the vast resources you possess to achieve the best result possible.

TURNING POINTS

1 Choose one aspect of your problem, a small aspect, and regard it as a difficult game that you wish to win.

2 Divide the game into opponents, challenges, abilities required, aims and any other components you can create.

3 Build up positive resources needed to improve your position in the game. Notice what you *learn* from your different attempts.

4 Take responsibility for putting into practice some different attitudes, approaches or responses to your problem.

5 Recognize that your problem is only a part of your life; don't let it take over completely.

27

Gleanings from experience

Some people have forty years of experience.
Others have one year of experience forty times.

During my years as a therapist I learnt a great deal from my clients. I've learnt what not to do, how to get in a muddle, how to continue going around in circles, how to become despondent and desperate.

I have also learnt about change, new guidelines, ways of learning and gaining from experience. I've learnt about hope, the strength of people to face their weaknesses, the risks necessary to overcome hurdles.

I have made small notes as I have learnt things and this chapter is a selection of brief points people have found helpful during the years. My advice is to look at them one at a time and check how they apply to you. If one is really significant write it down in a prominent place and turn it over in your mind again and again during the day. Check how you can change an inappropriate rule to one that is more suitable, more freeing and helpful in the direction you wish to go.

Don't be disheartened if change takes some time. One of the problems of books such as this is that readers get the idea that change occurs quickly and with ease. I can assure you that is *not* the case. Most people struggle, fail, feel it will never work, believe they have gone back to square one along the road to change. It is not easy, it is not simple and it is not quick, as a rule.

The following are a few thoughts that may be of use and a few guidelines that have proved helpful to those losing their way. They are only of value if you can put them into practice and not say to yourself how interesting they are as you close the book.

GLEANINGS FROM EXPERIENCE

- It is difficult to maintain relationships with others if you do not like yourself.
- Being assertive is very different from being aggressive.
- The words 'should' and 'shouldn't' imply someone else is running your life.
- In order to expand your world, to grow, it is necessary to take risks.
- It is better to have tried and failed than not to have tried at all.
- Growing up means taking responsibility.
- Relationship difficulties are often communication problems. Many barriers are caused by the belief that 'we are right and they are wrong' rather than 'we are different, what can I learn?'
- Problems are often challenges in disguise.
- Only give advice if you are offering new information.
- A person convinced against his will is of the same opinion still.
- If you are not a part of your own solutions you may

well be part of your own problems.
- 'I can't' is often another way of saying 'I won't', 'I'm too frightened to', 'I'd feel too guilty if . . .'
- We learn mostly from our own experiences. Those who go around in circles generally ignore their own positive experiences.
- To make decisions important for your personal growth use your intuition, deep feeling or bliss.
- Change is both complex and simple. Looking ahead at intended changes we see fear, failure and difficulty. Once change has occurred it seems simple on reflection. Like a trapeze artist, in order to grow you need to let go of what you are sure of, and grasp at uncertainty.
- Symptoms are generally *the result* of problems and not the problems themselves.
- We have a few basic patterns of behaviour and apply them to every situation we encounter. Increasing the number of patterns allows us a variety of choices.
- The map is not the territory. Our beliefs and reality are not the same. By failing to recognize the difference we remain in the same mould.
- Learning occurs on the cutting edge between the known and the unknown. In order to move into the unknown and claim it for ourselves we need to be open-minded, accept alternatives, take risks and face our fears. This process takes time, your own time.
- As a rule change is frightening. Anyone seeking change is accompanied by a part of themselves that wishes to stay the same.
- People cannot *make* you do, feel or act in any other way other than the way you *allow* them. Instead of 'he makes me angry' it is 'I allow him to make me angry'. Blaming others is a way of avoiding responsibility.
- A need to control often leads to situations where we are

out of control.

- Our attitudes and actions are the result of many different levels in our personality. Learning more about our deeper levels helps us to understand how we are what we are.
- Add fun as a companion to your journey through your life. The tasks are much lighter and the journey much easier.
- The Alcoholics Anonymous creed is:
    > God grant me the serenity to accept the things I cannot change,
    > Courage to change the things I can
    > And the wisdom to know the difference.

IN REALITY, IN YOUR OWN LIFE THERE ARE NO RULES, EXCEPT THIS ONE.

SOME GUIDELINES THAT MAY BE OF HELP

1) Live in the present
Too often we bemoan the past or anticipate worries in the future, directing our attention away from where life is – in the present.

2) Accept yourself as you are
(For the time being)
When we criticize, blame or judge ourselves, we colour the way we view the world.

3) Face your fears
Somehow avoidance causes the problem to persist, increase in magnitude or reappear at a most inconvenient time. As we face our fears we learn to grow and develop.

4) Have an attitude of 'what can I learn from situations'
This attitude means there are not successes and failures, but widening of horizons with experiences, whether positive or negative.

5) Make time for yourself
Most of us rush around always doing and trying. Being quiet and reflecting in a 'being' state restores the balance. Time for yourself should not be mistaken for selfishness.

6) Aim to be more aware, conscious
Most of our problems are caused by the unconscious mind – beyond our control. By bringing things to consciousness we gain the power over our behaviour.

7) Differentiate between 'problems' and 'nuisances'
If something is a *problem* we need to put effort into solving, changing or fixing it. Often it is a *nuisance* to put up with, accept or recognize.

8) Focus on your goal, your aim, what you hope to achieve
By being aware of your goal you can guide your feelings, attitudes and behaviour in the right direction; also be aware of 'the saboteur' inside trying to prevent change, trying to keep you as you are.

9) Understand your defence mechanisms
Make sure your defence mechanisms (attitudes, behaviour, habits) are *protecting* you from harm and not *preventing* you from enjoying yourself.

28

Conclusion

'There is greater pleasure in picking up a small pearl in an ash-can than in looking at a large one in a jeweller's window.'
Lin Yutang, *The Importance of Living*

Essentially the theme running through the pages is that we are all worthy individuals and that recognizing that fact ourselves and having others feel the same way, is extremely important for our well-being. Without it we head off on a merry-go-round search with resulting symptoms and discomfort.

Learning more about ourselves and the energy we are providing to maintain our problems is the first step towards getting off the merry-go-round. This book outlines a number of factors involved but is not, of course a 'cure'. Gathering some information about yourself from the words in the preceding pages will allow you to proceed, but motivation, commitment, effort and time need to follow before any change will result.

Many of the suggestions I have made will need the

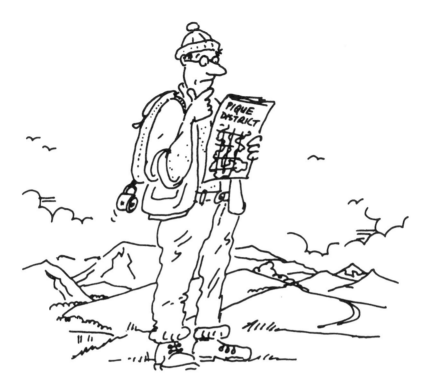

support and understanding of a therapist, friend or relative if they are to be put into effective practice. On the other hand it is possible to read this book, remark how interesting it is, yawn and continue on the merry-go-round.

At the conclusion of therapy, when clients have made the desired changes, I ask what has happened to achieve this result. Often we have been involved in many varied interactions – hypnosis, past life regression, visualization, etc.

What surprises me is that *every time* the response is the same. They ponder, reflect, look at the ceiling and say:

'You know Dr Roet, I think it was just having someone

listen to me and understand me without blame or criticism. That's what I believe helped me make to the changes.'

Life is a journey and the direction you take depends on the energy you provide and the aims you desire. I hope you have learnt something, however little, as you read these pages and that now, or in the future, they will provide the stepping stones for a healthier and happier pathway through your life. In a special book my daughter Sophie has for 'very important things' is a quote from Vita Sackville West's book *The Edwardians*:

'Life shapes itself, callous of our control but proves itself to have been wise at the end.'

PART 5

Your progress diary

Your name

....

Programme start date

....

Introduction

Congratulations! You have taken a major step in helping improve your health by buying the **Positive Action for Health and Wellbeing** programme. Unfortunately that is not enough. Research has shown that leaving it unread in your bookshelf produces no measurable benefit to your health. The next step is to read it – and read it in a way that the words on the page will be transformed into thoughts, attitudes and feelings. The **Progress Diary** and tapes are an additional aid to the main book, a little like a guide helping you over new territory. You will get the most from the **Positive Action for Health and Wellbeing** programme if you tailor the **Progress Diary** to your own specific needs.

The theme of the programme is that our mind and emotions play a major role in our health; by improving our attitudes and belief systems we will achieve improved health and play the 'game of life' with greater success. We learn so much from our parents and often the rules we inherit are unsuitable to our own personal needs. In order to achieve our own individual potential, we may need to 'relearn' many things so that our attitudes and actions are suitable for us in the present time.

Before you read or listen to anything, ask yourself the following questions:

- How bothered am I by my problems?
- Am I bothered enough to put time and effort into improving my life?
- Can I put up with things just as they are for the next 10 years?

Thirty years ago I decided to take up bee keeping. I bought a self-help book on bee keeping. The opening paragraph was:

'If when you think of bees you think of stings and feel frightened put the book down and proceed no further.'

I found that quite a shock from my new book. I *did* put the book down and thought long and hard about it. I came to the conclusion that I was scared of stings but *really* wanted the enjoyment of working with bees and collecting honey, so I read on.

I have had thirty years of wonderful experiences with bees. I've collected gallons of honey and made many friends. I've been stung many times, but have regarded the stings as minor inconveniences to me (and unfortunately death to the bee).

Your contribution will be time spent, mistakes made and effort invested. Again ask yourself the question:

'How bothered am I by my problems?'

In a song by Cat Stevens called *'Father and Son'*, the son says about his parents:

'If they were right I'd agree, but it's them they know not me.'

Our parents may have tried to help by advice and actions but 'it's them they know, not me' and the instructions given may well be unsuitable for our needs.

Being *your own* guide means you are aware of your difficulties and what you would like to achieve. This **Progress Diary** is aimed at helping you be a better guide to yourself. In order to benefit from it, you need to tailor the words on the pages and tapes to your own individual needs. The chapters are set out to illustrate different aspects of your mind and how it influences your life. Compare the test and case histories with your own specific needs.

To make the most of the **Positive Action for Health and Wellbeing** programme, follow a few basic rules:

1. Read the checklist carefully and apply the appropriate questions to your specific situation.
2. Think about the question and your response for some minutes, or hours, to allow it to be 'incubated'. This means that the question filters through different layers of the mind arousing other thoughts and questions. In this way you are making the most of the complex connections involved within conscious and unconscious parts of your mind.
3. Write down answers that seem suitable to your situation, and be aware of your attitude and behaviour relevant to this subject.
4. Have some quiet time, 5–10 minutes, to digest the subject, including self-praise for the time and effort you are putting in to achieve improvement.
5. Have a positive, non-judgmental attitude – 'What can I learn?' rather than 'Am I a success or failure?'
6. When situations arise that are related to a question, reflect on how you react to them and notice alternative ways of thinking or feeling about them.

There are two major components to life. One is *reality*, the other is our *belief* about this reality. For instance, someone who believes they are worthless will have much greater difficulties in life than someone who believes they are doing the best they can. It is the *belief* that guides us through life rather than *reality*. This **Progress Diary** is aimed at altering your beliefs about yourself and your world, so that your beliefs are more suitable for your needs.

Taking risks will help you learn much more than avoidance. People who use the concept 'anything for a peaceful life' have the least peaceful life of all.

Having quiet time for yourself every day is an essential component to better health. The pressure and racing of modern life creates many problems in our minds and bodies. Taking time to slow down is an important component of each day; it allows all the systems in the mind/body complex to perform at their best.

The two tapes provide a basis for this quiet time. Each side is twenty five minutes long and contains messages to produce relaxation and insight. Getting into the habit of listening to one side of a tape a day provides the benefits to the body that cleaning the teeth daily does for the gums and teeth. The messages on the tapes are absorbed much more easily and deeply because you are in a relaxed state. Storytelling has been the main method of communication for thousands of years. The story has a message wrapped up in an interesting container. We focus on the story and the unconscious receives the message; that is why folklore, bedtime stories and fables are so important.

Whilst listening to the tapes:

1. Allow yourself time so you are not concerned about what you are going to do next.
2. Be in a quiet place, undisturbed by people or phones.
3. Be in a passive mood, not an analytical one.
4. Be supported by a pillow or lying on the floor.
5. Listen to the tapes daily – not when you are tired, as you will go to sleep.

This **Progress Diary** is there to act as a guide. It is a series of questions to arouse interest in the specific aspects of that chapter. Tailor the questions to your own needs. It is *not* an exam, no one will be marking it, and it is a guide for *your* benefit to help you understand yourself better.

Being *aware* means you are in a much better place for improving your attitudes and thoughts, as they are all interlinked. There are five main components influencing you. They are all interlaced and being aware of these and their relationships means you are gaining control of your life. They are:

1. The environment – this means the places, situations and people who you are involved in your life – more specifically related to any problems you have.
2. Your thoughts about your problems and the environment.
3. Emotions resulting from your thoughts.
4. Your behaviour in response to the above three.
5. Physical reactions such as tension, insomnia, tiredness or pains, that are involved with the problem.

By *being aware* of these five components, and of the way they interact, and by asking yourself about them you are starting to run your life rather than being run by things. In any system it is worth 'trying the system' for a while and then having a breather, a rest to allow the information to 'incubate' in your mind. In this way you maintain interest and you benefit from the rest. You will know when it is time to have a break: maybe a week of working with the **Progress Diary**; perhaps one day on and one off. Work out the pattern that is best for you.

Reading a chapter of the book, then focussing on the **Progress Diary**, means you are tailoring the programme to your own specific needs. Don't hurry, take your time, proceed step by step. If you need more time to focus on one specific area then take it. It is not a race, it is a learning process and learning takes time – your own time.

It does work. I have seen it work many many times: people who put in more time and effort have better results than those that read as if it is something to do 'out there', an interesting read.

Treat this programme as a friend. The written and spoken words are there to help you – they come from twenty years of experience; it is now up to you to benefit from them.

All the best
Brian Roet

Chapter 1:
The long-term problem

CHECKLIST

1. Did you have 20 minutes quiet time yesterday?
   ☐ Yes ☐ No

2. Focus on one aspect of your problem and define it accurately.

3. Is it a real problem? ☐ Yes ☐ No

4. What measures have you taken to solve the problem?

5. Would 'acceptance' rather than fighting be a suitable solution? ☐ Yes ☐ No

6. List any of your attempts to solve the problem that may actually be maintaining it.

7. Are you avoiding or denying the problem? ☐ Yes ☐ No

8. (a) Could the problem be a message to you? ☐ Yes ☐ No
   (b) If so, what would the message be?

9. What can you learn from the problem:
   (a) about yourself

   (b) about your situation

10. List the strengths and abilities you would need to deal with the problem.

Chapter 2:
The patient

CHECKLIST

1. What role are your attitudes and beliefs playing in
   maintaining your problem?

   ....

   ....

2. Do you blame yourself or feel guilty about having
   your problem?

   □ Yes □ No

3. Has your energy been drained by worry, guilt or
   anxiety?

   □ Yes □ No

4. Check the list of characteristics and assess how many
   descriptions relate to you.

   ....

   ....

Chapter 3:
The need for a symptom

CHECKLIST

1. Have you spent twenty minutes quiet time in the last two days?

☐ Yes   ☐ No

2. In what way would your life be different when the symptoms are gone?

3. (a) Is your problem helping you avoid some aspects of your life?

☐ Yes   ☐ No

(b) If so, how could you change your attitude and face the problem rather than avoiding it?

4. List the benefits, the 'pay off' for your symptoms.

5. Where could you go to receive more help, support for your difficulties?

Chapter 4:
Challenging restricting beliefs

1. Make a list of the internal maps you are using to give you your attitudes and actions.

   _____

   _____

2. Are the maps:
   (a) useful?   ☐ Yes ☐ No
   (b) suitable?   ☐ Yes ☐ No
   (c) up-to-date?   ☐ Yes ☐ No

3. List some beliefs that are closer to reality (the territory) than the ones you have.

   _____

   _____

4. Do you use 'linking' of two facts with a 'because' to explain your attitudes and behaviour?

                                    ☐ Yes ☐ No

5. (a) Are you concerned what others think?

                                    ☐ Yes ☐ No

   (b) If yes do you believe it useful?

                                    ☐ Yes ☐ No

6. Make a list of new beliefs that would be releasing, supportive, and optimistic.

   _____

   _____

Chapter 5:
Negative self-talk

1. (a) Are you aware of your internal language?

   ☐ Yes ☐ No

   (b) If yes, what are you telling yourself?

   ....

   ....

   (c) Is it:
   - (i) optimistic   ☐ Yes ☐ No
   - (ii) pessimistic   ☐ Yes ☐ No
   - (iii) realistic   ☐ Yes ☐ No

2. (a) Do you have negative self-talk?   ☐ Yes ☐ No
   (b) If yes, is it in the form of :
   - (i) judging?   ☐ Yes ☐ No
   - (ii) criticism?   ☐ Yes ☐ No
   - (iii) blame?   ☐ Yes ☐ No
   - (iv) fear?   ☐ Yes ☐ No

3. Do you use words like should, must, ought to, in your internal language?

   ☐ Yes ☐ No

4. Do you have a 'catastrophiser' living in your head who creates concern by saying 'what if . . .' about a future event?

   ☐ Yes ☐ No

5. Write down what kind of internal guide you would like to have, who would be helpful and supportive.

   ....

   ....

6. Liking yourself is extremely important. Imagine you are going to tell someone about yourself. What would you say?

   ....

   ....

Chapter 6:
Imprinting – the fingerprints of fate

CHECKLIST

1. Have you spent some time and effort in the last two days to become more aware of the components of your problem?

    ☐ Yes   ☐ No

2. Write down the three components of an imprint.

    (a) _____

    (b) _____

    (c) _____

3. Was there a time in your life when an imprint may have happened to you?

    ☐ Yes   ☐ No

4. If yes, could the imprint be relevant to your present problem?

    ☐ Yes   ☐ No

5. If you have had an imprint affecting you then write down the situation in which it happened.

    ....

    ....

6. View the imprint from the perspective of the parent with all the power and control you have now and reduce its emotional effect by listing your strengths to deal with it.

    ....

    ....

Chapter 7:
Inner tension – a loss of power

1. List the signs you may have when you are tense – e.g. muscle tension, clenched fists, hunched shoulders.

2. Do your symptoms – high blood pressure, headaches, bowel problems – relate to tension?

☐ Yes ☐ No

3. (a) Do you have a good way of relaxing that you can practice to reduce tension?

☐ Yes ☐ No

(b) State what it is and how often you use it.

4. Do you have a massage to reduce muscle tension?

☐ Yes ☐ No

5. Conflict is when you (a) *wish* to do something but (b) believe that you *should* do something else.

List the areas in your life – work, relationships, hobbies – where conflicts occur.

Chapter 8:
The sinister partners of fear and guilt

CHECKLIST

1. Is fear a component of your problem? ☐ Yes ☐ No
2. If yes, state what your fear is.

   ....

3. Write down if the outcome you are frightened of is:
   (a) a possibility ☐ Yes ☐ No
   (b) a probability ☐ Yes ☐ No
4. If you are frightened of something happening, look at your experiences and write down the likelihood of it happening.

   ....

5. If you have fear about something, write down the *actual* feelings that occur in your body which make up the feeling called *fear*.

   ....

   ....

6. Is guilt a feeling involved with your problem?
   ☐ Yes ☐ No
7. If yes, are you using self-punishment to justify the guilt?
   ☐ Yes ☐ No
8. Is it reasonable:
   (a) to continue punishing yourself? ☐ Yes ☐ No
   (b) to assume you can stop the self-punishment?
   ☐ Yes ☐ No
9. (a) Are the situations in the past responsible for your guilt?
   ☐ Yes ☐ No
   (b) If so, look back on them from today's perspective and assess if punishment is still warranted.
10. Each day make a commitment to face up to any fear or guilt that may be related to your problem. Be kind, caring and understanding to yourself, so you will be free to deal with life's difficulties.

Chapter 9:
Mad, bad or misunderstood?

1. A good relationship is defined as each partner having his or her needs met. When you have a difference of opinion with your partner, do you take an attitude of:

   (a) I'm right and they are wrong   ☐ Yes   ☐ No

   (b) It is their fault the difference of opinion occurred

        ☐ Yes   ☐ No

   (c) We are just different, not better or worse than each other   ☐ Yes   ☐ No

   (d) I always get it wrong   ☐ Yes   ☐ No

2. (a) Do you use the words should/shouldn't when discussing a difference of opinion with each other?

        ☐ Yes   ☐ No

   (b) Try and converse without using should/shouldn't as they are judging words and imply a moralising attitude.

3. (a) Do you use criticism as a way of expressing a differing point of view?

        ☐ Yes   ☐ No

   (b) If 'yes', what other ways could you state your differences?

   ....

   ....

Chapter 10:
The doctor's role

CHECKLIST

1. Chronic conditions have psychological as well as physical conditions.
   (a) List the psychological components of your problem.

   ....

   ....

   (b) In what ways could you minimise these components?

   ....

   ....

2. (a) Does your doctor understand your condition?

   ☐ Yes   ☐ No

   (b) Do you find that your doctor is a good listener?

   ☐ Yes   ☐ No

   (c) Do you seek other people to act as listeners for your complaints?

   Friends?   ☐ Yes   ☐ No

   Partners?   ☐ Yes   ☐ No

   Alternative therapists?   ☐ Yes   ☐ No

3. Liking yourself is one of the basic attitudes that helps you through life. Spend a few minutes praising some of the things you have done in the last few days.

Chapter 11:
The importance of understanding

1. As understanding yourself is so very important, write a brief description of whom you believe you are – attitudes, beliefs, emotions.

   ....

   ....

2. As well as understanding yourself it is important to accept yourself 'warts and all'. Are you able to say: 'I accept myself'?   ☐ Yes   ☐ No

3. Choose someone close to you – partner, parent or child.
   (a) Do you understand them?   ☐ Yes   ☐ No
   (b) How could you learn to understand them more?

   ....

4. Thoughts, feeling and behaviour are linked. Focus on an incident that happened recently and write the connection between the three components of your life.
   My thought was:

   ....

   which caused the feeling of:

   ....

   which resulted in the behaviour:

   ....

5. (a) State any negative thoughts that continually occur causing adverse feelings and behaviour.

   ....

   (b) Write down alternative thoughts that may result in improved behaviour.

   ....

Chapter 12:
Fixation on the physical

CHECKLIST

1. State the physical component of your problem (feelings and symptoms).

2. Write down what psychological factors may be involved:
   (a) as a *cause* of that feeling

   (b) as a *result* of that feeling

3. Learning to like yourself, accepting yourself, is a major component of feeling better.
   Write an 'identikit' list that describes who you are e.g. the physical, emotional, attitudes, beliefs that you hold.

   Would you be able to state that you accept yourself for the time being?

4. Are situations, attitudes, beliefs that affect your symptoms:
   (a) in the past   ☐ Yes ☐ No
   (b) in the present   ☐ Yes ☐ No
   (c) in the future   ☐ Yes ☐ No
5. Are your symptoms related to:
   (a) situations you are in   ☐ Yes ☐ No
   (b) other people's attitudes   ☐ Yes ☐ No
   (c) your attitude towards yourself   ☐ Yes ☐ No

Chapter 13:
How the other half lives – the unconscious

1. How would you describe the circumstances?

....

....

2. How are you aware of its existence?

....

....

3. State ways in which the unconscious mind influences:
   (a) your life

   ....

   (b) your symptoms

   ....

4. (a) Is your unconscious active while you are asleep?

   ☐ Yes   ☐ No

   (b) If yes, does that actually influence how you feel?

   ☐ Yes   ☐ No

5 List any of your symptoms that may be related to conscious activity.

....

....

Chapter 14:
Different levels of controlling behaviour

CHECKLIST

1. Sit quietly for a few minutes. Imagine your mind consisting of different levels. Take some time to allow yourself to explore the levels and learn about their activity.
   Are some levels more helpful than others?

   ☐ Yes   ☐ No

2. Every few nights spend some time drifting down to levels you find helpful and appropriate for you.

Chapter 15:
It's about time

CHECKLIST

1. Time is a factor in many of our experiences. Make sure you have quiet time in the next few days to balance other activities.

2. Become aware of your 'timing'. Imagine a metronome inside your mind. Would it be going fast or slowly? Is your partner's timing the same as yours?

3. (a) Are you a future worrier?   ☐ Yes   ☐ No

   (b) Is your mind constantly asking 'what if?'?

   ☐ Yes   ☐ No

   (c) Or are you living in the past with the question, 'if only' directing your attitudes and behaviour?

   ☐ Yes   ☐ No

4. What percentage of the day are you in the present, in the 'here and now'?

5. Give yourself some time to reflect on the last 24 hours with an attitude of 'what can I learn from what happened?'.

Chapter 16:
The diversionary tactics of stress

CHECKLIST

1. (a) Make a list of 5 situations in your life where stress plays a major role.

   (1) ....

   (2) ....

   (3) ....

   (4) ....

   (5) ....

   (b List the symptoms or attitudes resulting from these stressful situations.

   ....

   ....

2. What role does stress play in your problem, either:

   (a) as a cause factor

   ....

   ....

   (b) resulting from the problem

   ....

   ....

3. (a) Are you a mind-reader concerned about what other people think?

   ☐ Yes   ☐ No

   (b) If yes, focus on becoming aware of when you are 'mind-reading' and take steps to reduce it.

4. Think about your problem being a message to inform you. What would the message be? Is this message suitable and up-to-date?

5. Make a commitment to do a relaxation exercise in the next 24 hours.

Chapter 17:
A breath of fresh air – hyperventilation

CHECKLIST

1. Hyperventilation is often an underlying cause of symptoms. Sit comfortably with one hand on your chest and the other on your abdomen. Breathe naturally and notice which hand is moving more.
2. If your chest hand is moving more than the one on your abdomen, you are likely to be a hyperventilator.
3. Check with the symptoms list to assess how many you have.
4. If you are a hyperventilator, make a commitment to see a physiotherapist to help improve your breathing.

Chapter 18:
How are your feelings?

CHECKLIST

1. Make a list of:

   (a) the most common feelings you have

   ....

   (b) the feelings that cause you the most bother

   ....

2. (a) What feelings do you have that indicate you don't like/ accept yourself?

(b) What feelings would you replace them with in order to feel better about yourself?

3. Think of an incident that happened today that was associated with a feeling:
    (a) give the feeling a label

    (b) whereabouts in your body was it?

    (c) acknowledge that it was alright to have the feeling
    (d) express the feeling by telling someone else or writing it down

    (e) 'go into' the feeling to explore what message it was sending you

4. Build up a store of positive feelings and *anchor* them by clenching your hand as you experience the feeling.
5. Are you:
    (a) more relaxed

    (b) more emotional

    (c) balanced between the two?

Chapter 19:
Analyzing the 'parts'

1. Think of yourself as made up of different parts, characters. Write a list of the main internal characters influencing your life.

   ....

   ....

2. Sit quietly for 10 minutes and imagine these parts as if they are individual people living inside you and influencing your attitudes and behaviour.

3. (a) Would you like to introduce any new parts who would be beneficial to the way you think, act or feel?

   ....

   ....

   (b) Are there any parts you would like to reduce in size and sound so their influence is diminished?

   ....

   ....

4. Do some situations trigger off a specific part of you to respond?

   ....

   ....

Chapter 20:
The real me

1. The concept 'the real me' is very helpful in distinguishing 'you' as a person and the 'you' that has been covered by layers of experience.

    (a) Spend some time thinking about 'the real me' – your genuine beliefs, attitudes and behaviour.

    (b) Compare the person within you as you act and react on a daily basis.

    How much difference is there between (a) and (b)?

2. On what areas are you 'playing a role' that differs from your true nature?

    (a) at work   ☐ Yes ☐ No
    (b) at relationships   ☐ Yes ☐ No
    (c) within the family   ☐ Yes ☐ No
    (d) in leisure activities   ☐ Yes ☐ No

253

Chapter 21:
The memory lingers on

1. Memories influence our attitudes, behaviour, the way we react to different situations. What role do memories of past traumas play in influencing your attitudes and confidence?

2. In the Chapter there are six steps to improve the memory.
   (a) Choose a past experience that is reducing your confidence.
   (b) Go through the 6 steps to lower the effect the memory is having on your present behaviour.

3. (a) Choose a 'future memory' that has associated fears and doubts.
   (b) Go through the 6 steps to improve the future memory so you feel confident and positive about the future events.

4. Each day make a commitment to change a negative memory into a positive one.

Chapter 22:
Creative visualization

CHECKLIST

1. The way we know the world is through self-talk, our internal tape recordings, visualizations, pictures we create in the mind, feelings, emotions from past experiences.

   Choose a feeling that is troubling you.

   (a) Find out where in your body it is situated.

   (b) Imagine what it looks like – colour, shape, whether small or moving, size.

2. (a) Think of a feeling you would rather have than the one that is troubling you.

   (b) Imagine what this new feeling would look like.

   (c) Change the troubled picture into the positive one.

   (d) Notice the change in feeling.

Chapter 23:
The forgotten child within

CHECKLIST

1. One of the most important and powerful techniques in therapy is 'the child within'. Consider some of your actions as if they are coming from the child within.

2. Spend some quiet time with the 'child'. Have an attitude of listening, caring and understanding towards the child; help him/her to feel better. Realise that things change, situations pass and improvement occurs.

3. Help to reduce fear, guilt, anger or shame that the child feels due to their situation. Give praise and support to confidence and acceptance replacing the negative self-doubts.

Chapter 24:
Panning for gold

CHECKLIST

1. Our attitudes to experiences play a major role in how we enjoy life. Noticing good things that happen, pleasures we gain through the day adds 'sugar to the cake'.

   Before you go to bed spend 10 minutes reviewing the day with a positive attitude. Note only the things you enjoyed, that gave you pleasure – however small.

2. As you go to sleep, allow these 'specks of gold' to drift around in your mind so they focus your dreams on success throughout the night.

Chapter 25:
Alternative choices

1. One way of looking at our progress through life is that we develop more choices. The more choice we have the easier it is to find a suitable solution.

   Look at a problem you have and list *all* the choices available to you.

2. Make a list of what is preventing you attempting these choices.

3. Are the preventative factors:

   (a) coming from external sources?

   (b) related to your attitudes and emotions?

4. Observe whether your methods of 'attempting change' are actually 'preventing change'.

5. List ways you could add humour to your methods of overcoming your problem.

257

Chapter 26:
Taking responsibility

1. Different aspects of your problems may be regarded as challenges. By learning more about them you will be able to deal with them and learn in the process.

2. Take one aspect of your problem and divide it into:

   (a) challenge required to deal with

   (b) abilities needed

   (c) desired outcome

   (d) time necessary to achieve outcome

3. Make a commitment to put these theoretical concepts into practice. Take responsibility to complete this by a certain time.

4. Be aware that the problem is only part of your life. Prevent it taking over your thoughts and feelings.

Chapter 27:
Gleanings from experience

In order to 'play the game of life' by the most suitable rules a few guidelines may help. In order to be of more use these need to be 'taken on board' rather than read as interesting items.

Focus on one point a day and remind yourself by repeating or writing it somewhere it will be noticed.

1. Live in the present.
2. Accept yourself as you are (for the time being).
3. Face your fears rather than using avoidance.
4. Have an attitude of 'what can I learn' from situations.
5. Have quiet time each day for yourself.
6. Aim to be more aware of yourself, thoughts, feelings and surroundings.
7. Change 'problems' into 'nuisances'.
8. Be aware when it is suitable to 'accept' as well as when it is suitable to 'fix'.

Reading List

Alman, Brian and Lambron, Peter, *Self-Hypnosis: The complete manual for health and self-image*, Souvenir Press, 1993

Austin, Valerie, *Self-Hypnosis*, Thorsons, 1994

Bach, Richard, *Illusions*, Pan Books, 1978

Balint, Michael, *The Doctor, His Patient and the Illness*, Pitman, 1964

Charles, Rachel, *Your Mind's Eye*, Piatkus, 2000

Dainow, Sheila, *Be Your Own Counsellor*, Piatkus, 1997

Gendlin, Eugene T., *Focussing*, Bantam New Age, 1978

Harrison, Eric, *How Meditation Heals*, Piatkus, 2000

Harrison, John, *Love Your Disease, It's Keeping You Healthy*, Angus & Robertson, 1984

Hesse, Herman, *Siddhartha*, Picador, 1973

Kopp, Sheldon, *The Hanged Man*, Sheldon Press, 1981

Linn, Denise, *Past Lives, Present Dreams*, Piatkus, 1994

Roet, Brian, *The Confidence to Be Yourself*, Piatkus, 1998

Roet, Brian, *Understanding Hypnosis*, Piatkus, 2000

Stuart, Cristina, *Speak for Yourself*, Piatkus, 2000

Sweet, Corinne, *Overcoming Addiction*, Piatkus, 1999

Weekes, Claire, *Self-help for your nerves*, Thorsons, 1995

Werbach, Melvyn R., *Third Line Medicine*, Arkana, 1986

Have you found **Positive Action for Health and Wellbeing** practical and useful? If so, you may be interested in other books from Class Publishing.

High blood pressure at your fingertips
NEW SECOND EDITION! £14.99
Dr Julian Tudor Hart with Dr Tom Fahey

The authors use all their years of experience as blood pressure experts to answer your questions on high blood pressure.

Diabetes at your fingertips
FOURTH EDITION! £14.99
Professor Peter Sonksen,
Dr Charles Fox and Sister Sue Judd

461 questions on diabetes are answered clearly and accurately – the ideal reference book for everyone with diabetes.

> 'I have no hesitation in commending this book' – *Sir Harry Secombe CBE, President of the British Diabetic Association*

Heart health at your fingertips
NEW SECOND EDITION! £14.99
Dr Graham Jackson

This practical handbook, written by a leading cardiologist, answers all your questions about heart conditions.

> 'Contains the answers the doctor wishes he had given if only he'd had the time.' – *Dr Thomas Stuttaford,* The Times

Cancer information at your fingertips
NEW THIRD EDITION! £14.99
Val Speechley and Maxine Rosenfield

Recommended by the Cancer Research Campaign, this book provides straightforward and positive answers to all your questions about cancer.

Alzheimer's at your fingertips
Harry Cayton, Dr Nori Graham,
Dr James Warner £14.99

At last – a book that tells you everything you need to know about Alzheimer's and other dementias.

> 'an invaluable contribution to understanding all forms of dementia.' – *Dr Jonathan Miller CBE, President, Alzheimer's Disease Society*

Stop that heart attack!
NEW SECOND EDITION! £14.99
Dr Derrick Cutting

The easy, drug-free and medically accurate way to cut your risk of having a heart attack dramatically.

Even if you already have heart disease, you can halt and even reverse its progress by following Dr Cutting's simple stpes. Don't be a victim – take action NOW!

Parkinson's at your fingertips
NEW SECOND EDITION! £14.99
Dr Marie Oxtoby
and Professor Adrian Williams

Full of practical help and advice for people with Parkinson's disease and their families. This book gives you the information and the confidence to tackle the challenges that PD presents.

> 'An unqualified success'–*Dr Andrew Lees, Consultant Neurologist, The National Hospital for Neurology and Neurosurgery*

Allergies at your fingertips
Dr Joanne Clough £14.99

At last – sensible practical advice on allergies from an experienced medical expert.

> 'An excellent book which deserves to be on the bookshop of every family.' – *Dr Csaba Rusznak, Medical and Scientific Director, British Allergy Foundation*

Asthma at your fingertips
NEW THIRD EDITION! £14.99
Dr Mark Levy, Professor Sean Hilton
and Greta Barnes MBE

This book shows you how to keep your asthma – or your family's asthma – under control, making it easier to live a full, happy and healthy life.

> 'This book gives you the knowledge. Don't limit yourself.' – *Adrian Moorhouse MBE, Olympic Gold Medallist*

Positive Action for Health and Wellbeing

In this programme, Dr Brian Roet explains simply and clearly about the positive steps you can take to promote your own health and wellbeing.

Positive Action for Health and Wellbeing includes:

- **Practical guide**
- **Your progress diary**
- **Double cassette pack**

Using straightforward, easy and effective methods, the author shows you tried and tested steps to better health and self-esteem. Armed with this encouraging and empowering package, you can overcome difficult problems, allievate pain, reduce stress and tackle any fears and phobias you may have.

Positive Action for Health and Wellbeing shows you how to:

- Increase your self-confidence!
- Break free from your current problems and worries!
- Make positive steps to start afresh with a new zest for life!
- Enjoy the process of unlocking your potential!
- Improve your health and wellbeing!

In his complete programme, Dr Roet reinforces the practical messages in this book with a comprehensive double cassette pack, and personal progress diary.

Positive Action for Health and Wellbeing
NEW! Only £29.99!

The complete step-by-step programme to take control of your life and your health.
Includes:

- Practical guide
- Your progress diary
- Double cassette pack

Each item in the programme is also available separately:

Positive Action for Health and Wellbeing
NEW! Only £14.99!
The practical guide to taking control of your life and your health

Positive Action for Health and Wellbeing
NEW! Only £2.99!
Your progress diary

Positive Action for Health and Wellbeing
NEW! Only £13.99!
Double cassette pack

PLEASE TURN OVER FOR DETAILS OF HOW TO ORDER ☛

PRIORITY ORDER FORM

Cut out or photocopy this form and send it (post free in the UK) to:

Class Publishing Priority Service   Tel: 01752 202301
FREEPOST (PAM 6219)   Fax: 01752 202333
Plymouth PL6 7ZZ

Please send me urgently   *Post included*
(tick boxes below)   *price per copy (UK only)*

☐ Positive Action for Health and Wellbeing: complete programme	£32.99
☐ Positive Action for Health and Wellbeing: practical guide	£17.99
☐ Positive Action for Health and Wellbeing: progress diary	£4.99
☐ Positive Action for Health and Wellbeing: cassette pack	£16.99
☐ High blood pressure at your fingertips	£17.99
☐ Diabetes at your fingertips	£17.99
☐ Heart health at your fingertips	£17.99
☐ Stop that heart attack!	£17.99
☐ Parkinson's at your fingertips	£17.99
☐ Allergies at your fingertips	£17.99
☐ Asthma at your fingertips	£17.99
☐ Cancer information at your fingertips	£17.99
☐ Alzheimer's at your fingertips	£17.99

TOTAL _____

Easy ways to pay

Cheque: I enclose a cheque payable to Class Publishing for £ _____

Credit card: Please debit my   ☐ Access   ☐ Visa   ☐ Amex   ☐ Switch

Number _____ Expiry date _____

Name _____

My address for delivery is _____

_____

Town _____ County _____ Postcode _____

Telephone number (in case of query) _____

Credit card billing address if different from above _____

_____

Town _____ County _____ Postcode _____

Class Publishing's guarantee: remember that if, for any reason, you are not satisfied with these books, we will refund all your money, without any questions asked. Prices and VAT rates may be altered for reasons beyond our control.